Managing High Security Psychiatric Care

Forensic Focus

This series, now edited by Gwen Adshead, takes the currently crystallising field of Forensic Psychotherapy as its focal point, offering a forum for the presentation of theoretical and clinical issues. It will also embrace such influential neighbouring disciplines as language, law, literature, criminology, ethics and philosophy, as well as psychiatry and psychology, its established progenitors.

Forensic Psychotherapy
Crime, Psychodynamics and the Offender Patient
Edited by Christopher Cordess and Murray Cox
ISBN 1 85302 240 3 (two hardback volumes)
ISBN 1 85302 634 4 (one volume paperback))
Forensic Focus 1

The Cradle of Violence
Essays on Psychiatry, Psychoanalysis and Literature
Stephen Wilson
ISBN 1 85302 306 X
Forensic Focus 2

Psychiatric Assessment
Pre and Post Admission Assessment
Valerie Anne Brown
ISBN 1 85302 575 5
Forensic Focus 8

A Practical Guide to Forensic Psychotherapy
Edited by Estela V. Welldon and Cleo Van Velsen
Forewords by Fiona Caldicott, DBE and Helena Kennedy QC
ISBN 1 85302 389 2
Forensic Focus 3

Challenges in Forensic Psychotherapy
Edited by Hjalmar van Marle and Wilma van den Berg
ISBN 1 85302 419 8
Forensic Focus 5

Remorse and Reparation
Edited by Murray Cox
ISBN 85302 451 1 (hardback)
ISBN 85302 452 X (paperback)
Forensic Focus 7

Forensic Focus 9

Managing High Security Psychiatric Care

Edited by Charles Kaye and Alan Franey

Jessica Kingsley Publishers
London and Philadelphia

First published in the United Kingdom in 1998 by
Jessica Kingsley Publishers Ltd
116 Pentonville Road,
London N1 9JB, England
and
325 Chestnut Street,
Philadelphia, PA19106, USA

Copyright © 1998 Jessica Kingsley Publishers

Library of Congress Cataloging in Publication Data
A CIP catalogue record for this book is available from the Library of Congress

British Library Cataloguing in Publication Data
A CIP catalogue record for this book is available from the British Library

ISBN 1 85302 581 X (pb)
ISBN 1 85302 582 8 (hb)

Printed and Bound in Great Britain by
Athenaeum Press, Gateshead, Tyne and Wear

Contents

Figures

Tables

To Hilary and Lesley
who have shared the journey

O the mind, mind has mountains, cliffs of fall
Frightful, sheer, no-man-fathomed. Hold them cheap
May who ne'er hung there. Nor does long our small
Durance deal with that steep of deep.

Gerard Manley Hopkins

Acknowledgements

No enterprise like this is achieved without considerable help from many people. We have been very conscious of imposing on colleagues and friends to check recollections and test perceptions. Needless to say we alone take responsibility for the views expressed in our chapters and for whatever errors and misconceptions they may contain.

We have many people to thank; it is a pleasant task to acknowledge their help and enthusiasm.

Jackie Hayward has worked closely with us throughout the preparation of the book; she has shared much of the hard work which lies behind the creation of the final text and we would like to acknowledge her invaluable contribution.

Particular mention must also be made of the late Dr Murray Cox who supported, with his usual gusto, the idea of this book and who commented helpfully and perceptively on several early drafts. Our sorrow is that this fruitful collaboration was cut short by his sudden death.

Martin Butwell, from the Professorial Unit at Broadmoor Hospital, has gone out of his way to be helpful in supplying statistics and pointing out the significance of patterns emerging. We have included some simple tables in Appendix 2 and included some important references in our main text. We know that it is the intention of Professor Taylor and Martin Butwell to publish a more comprehensive statistical review which will be welcomed by all workers in this field.

Our librarians have been patient, resourceful and charming: we thank Alison Farrar, Judy Phillips and Caroline Reynolds at Broadmoor Hospital and Brenda Goddard at the Royal Hampshire County Hospital, Winchester.

Many people have commented on drafts and offered valuable advice and assistance. Among those we would like particularly to mention: Georgina Allnutt, Dorothy Barrett, Steve Brewster, Dr Julian Candy, Margaret Cudmore, Sheila Drew Smith, Dr Chandra Ghosh, Jo Green, Roger Hinton, Tony Lingiah, John Lynch, Brian Johnson, Joy Kinsley, Linda Lowe, Les Martin, Nuala O'Brien, Sir James Savile, Joanna Sheehan, Professor Pamela Taylor and Alison Webster. We would also like to thank Cathy Nightingale for her very professional work in realising our vague ideas for the front and back covers of the book.

Charles Kaye and Alan Franey

PART 1

Introduction

CHAPTER 1

Fundamental Themes

Charles Kaye and Alan Franey

INTRODUCTION

This book looks at the recent developments in this country's high security psychiatric service as currently provided in the three Special Hospitals, Ashworth, Broadmoor and Rampton. It describes those hospitals and ways in which changes and improvements have been introduced and consolidated. It acknowledges that this is work in progress but claims that significant advances have been made over the past decade.

Although contributors have been encouraged to describe this process from their own point of view – as doctor, chaplain, patient or as involved outsider – the overall perspective is that of the manager. In this context, the manager is taken to be the leader, the one who indicates the direction of progress and encourages the team towards that goal. This is totally different from the role and scope of the administrator who formerly featured within the special hospital hierarchy. No claims are made that only managers can be leaders; that would obviously be absurd. However, we contend that at this juncture of the service's life, the leadership task was given to managers specifically and deliberately. The record that follows shows how they set about that work with clinical colleagues and illustrates some of the successes and some of the failures. It is an honest account, not designed as a paean of self-praise.

It aims to illuminate a notorious, but little understood world, to allow its complexities and paradoxes to be realised and to share its tensions. The work and the institutions are far removed from most people's experience, even many of those working in health and criminal justice.

As essential preparation for the later chapters, we are setting out some of the themes that dominate the special hospitals and the service they provide. These are matters which reoccur continually within the individual contributions but, of course, from different perspectives. Each in turn alters the view and it is often difficult to retain the overall context.

To provide the context we have divided our broad survey into five areas (see Figure 1.1).

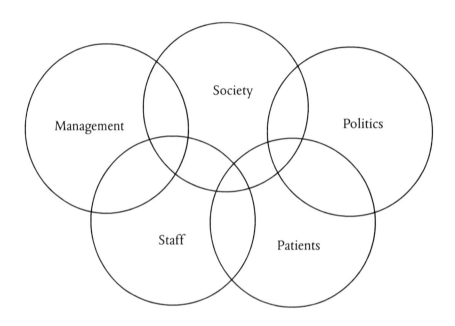

Figure 1.1 : Interlocking worlds in high security

Such distinctions will help to clarify but they can also mislead. As a cautionary note it is worth stating that our experience not only shows that all these areas interconnect and interrelate but also that, on occasion, the relationship may be a chain reaction which, with bewildering speed, accelerates to the point of explosion. We describe a volatile world.

SOCIETY

As a society we are deeply ambivalent about care and therapy for those whose illness has expressed itself in violence and anti-social behaviour. The ordered and measured view of those for whom the high security service exists is expressed by Sir John Wood:

> If responsibility cannot be plainly determined, the decision as to whether there should be treatment or punishment is equally uncertain. It is small

wonder that there is a feeling that many are punished, particularly by imprisonment, who should not be, and others are given treatment without clear evidence that this will prove to be of benefit. It is only possible to conclude that the whole question of responsibility and the legitimacy of the reaction of the state to deviancy is full of uncertainties and problems. (Wood 1995)

An alternative response to the same dilemma comes from a different source:

Broadmoor is not just a hospital with bars. It is a prison. And should be run like one. (*The Mail on Sunday* 1997)

This view is broadcast with considerably more decibels and is a regular theme for much of the media for whom 'bad' is far better copy than 'mad'.

Thus illustrated is an essential tension between fairness and fear. There is acceptance in the law and institutions of the country of the only partly understood connections between mental illness and aberrant behaviour. As a compassionate society we make provision and hope to offer individuals the chance of treatment, rehabilitation and reinstatement. As individuals making up that society we feel fear and resent the risks that the compassion requires. What is risk to the professional is danger to the general public.

The media reflect most clearly this ambivalence but it sits everywhere, in the wider NHS and indeed, on occasion, in the staff of the hospitals themselves. It is irresolvable because it represents what is not understood and cannot be explained by lawyer, reporter or psychiatrist. But it does mean that the hospitals and their staff work with little public support or understanding and, often, with public criticism. Several years ago a patient escaped from a working party outside the hospital's perimeter; he was close to transfer and that amount of freedom was thought a reasonable risk. A few days later the wife of the nurse in charge of the working party was confronted in her local supermarket by an angry neighbour condemning her husband for endangering the neighbourhood. The effect of such pressures on staff is not difficult to imagine. Implicitly it supports the custodial and denies the therapeutic. By their very existence such forces contribute to the separation, the isolation of staff from their fellow citizens. At the height of the publicity following the first Ashworth Inquiry, some staff would not willingly admit where they worked, denying their very purpose.

The work is in the public eye and little distinction is made in that glare between taking measured risks, making mistakes or even unfounded rumours. All are likely to be pounced upon, headlined, condemned and abandoned before any response or evaluation can properly be made. An unforgiving public is impatient with explanation and justification. But the responsibility remains and with it the requirement to treat and to respond to individual needs.

At a national level there are formal mechanisms for sharing the responsibility; the sophistication and size of a national bureaucracy can apportion and absorb conflicting needs. So the Home Office, in its control of restricted patients[1] (whose number is steadily increasing), can be the public's watchdog, both examining and sharing the doctors' decisions on the futures of individual patients. The doctor proposes; the Home Office decides. Often that appears to health staff to present an additional obstacle with dark mutterings in the special hospitals about 'unwritten tariffs'. In practice it is the bureaucratic check to reduce risk and guard public safety. Is it surprising that it is exercised with caution and thus geared to public concern and public outcry?

This is not a phenomenon confined to forensic psychiatry. At a conference of scientists held at the Royal Society in March 1996 (*Nature* 1996) on the handling of risks there was consensus on the principle that public perceptions must be included in the assessment of risks: 'We did not grasp the very different way the consumer sees risk', said the chairman of the UK Advisory Committee on Novel Foods and Processes.

POLITICS

In one sense the Department of Health and the Home Office can be seen as representing the two poles of the special hospital world, therapy and security. The need to care and the need to guard must co-exist at every level. Reality, and public opinion, suggests that the latter function will, on occasion, outweigh the former, as when the Home Secretary abruptly stopped special hospital rehabilitation trips because of public concern about 'soft' policies for home trips for prisoners. At best the two Departments collaborated fruitfully – as with the creation of the Special Hospital Service Authority (SHSA) itself. This adroit move in 1989 fulfilled a number of useful objectives:

1. It brought in management skills and discipline where they were much needed (HAS 1988).

2. It was within the Next Steps programme, which devolved central government functions to other bodies (but still maintaining significant control politically).

3. It removed over 3000 staff from the Civil Service payroll by making them employees of a quango.

---

1   The Home Office has the legal duty to make the final decision on hospital leave or transfer recommendations for some patients; they are therefore 'restricted'. The population detained in hospitals at the end of 1996 was 2586 – higher than in any of the previous ten years (Home Office 1997).

4.   It distanced central government and ministers from some of the worst pressures of being directly accountable for everything in the special hospital service.

5.   It allowed the new managers more freedom to lead and change; by the same token it offered more space to the hospitals in their clinical role.

Of course, between central government and their quangos, the boundaries are written in sand and the tide of events can shift and even obliterate them. The Michael Howard/Derek Lewis distinction between policy and operations is a nice example. It sounds an attractive demarcation but it is impossible to separate them fully; their real relationship is reciprocal. Management is just as likely to be the architect (even if often anonymous) of policy as the Secretary of State, for example, is to dictate who watches TV in their cells. The management of this uncertainty and shift in a health authority with national responsibilities is a key part of the work of the Chairman and Chief Executive. Acute crisis can intervene and politicians take over – as with the Ashworth Inquiry and the escape from Broadmoor Hospital in the early 1990s. But such extremes can usually be endured and weathered without having to jettison key management objectives. Indeed the imperatives of crisis will often enable the good manager to advance other objectives – after the Ashworth Inquiry report some changes were quickly made that would have taken much longer in other circumstances.

Much of the relationship rests on personality and confidence; certainly open conflict produces casualties and there the managers' armour is considerably lighter than that of other participants.

In the context of politics, there can be no pure managerial objectives or territory; all is subject to political and public influence (the one often reflecting the other). The manager is always politically accountable and must be prepared to explain, persuade, concede and persist.

PATIENTS

As Professor Elaine Murphy comments:

> The most striking feature of the special hospital patients is the enormous diversity of their individual needs for specific therapeutic interventions...
> (Murphy 1996)

One way of describing the management task would be as the creation of an environment where patients are recognised as individuals, not diagnoses or 'index offences'[2], and receive care and treatment appropriate to their needs. More usually an institution organises its residents in patterns which help it to run

---

2   Particular offence(s) for which a patient is detained.

smoothly (and often cheaply). The SHSA's task was to reverse that relationship: to revolve the institution around the individual. That is a task still incomplete. Indeed it must be questionable whether any institutions as large as the special hospitals can really be sensitised to the extent of providing over 400 patients with personally fitting programmes. While size offers variety in terms of facilities and therapies, it also imposes conformity in terms of routines and practices.

The painful process of emphasising the individual has left scars and produced harsh dilemmas. Certainly for many staff the emphasis on patients as people having rights was felt as a direct threat to their own standing. Within the new complaints system the recognition of the potential validity of evidence from patients was seen as a direct devaluation of the importance of staff. Again the creation of a patients' advocacy service and the complementary Patients' Council was regarded as the 'handing over' of a measure of control to the patient population. This protest reached such a crescendo in 1997 that it provoked a direct political intervention with the appointment of a review team to assess the reality of that impression at Broadmoor Hospital. They reached the following conclusion:

> Allegations have been made that the Patients' Council within Broadmoor are unduly influencing the management of the hospital. The Review Team did not find any evidence that this is true and can categorically state that the Patients' Council does not run Broadmoor.

> In summary, Broadmoor has undertaken a vast programme of change over recent years. From a background of institutional custodial care, it has been actively moving towards the development of a service which seeks to provide therapeutic care within a secure setting. It cannot be stressed enough that it is the excellent work of clinical, professional and support staff that has enabled this process of change to be undertaken without compromise of public safety. However, these changes also bring with them elements of disquiet and concern. The concerns relate to the ability of staff to retain security in an environment where therapeutic care approaches challenge previously acceptable practices. (*Donovan Report* 1997)

It might seem obvious that patients' 'rights' were set within a clear context which also set goals and drew boundaries. They were part of the philosophy of growth within control. To staff who had seen order and control as ends in themselves it was a challenge, both to their experience and to their view of the patient. Some reacted defensively, some overcompensated, sulkily asserting they no longer had authority over the patients. And some patients were quick to take advantage of such a withdrawal. Giving patients rights did not necessarily make them responsible individuals nor relieve them of their psychosis, nor expunge the behaviour that had caused them to be admitted originally. As with so many issues in the hospitals, action to introduce desirable change had strong reciprocal effects elsewhere within the institution.

Importantly, this emphasis on rights recognised another essential feature of the patients' world: their vulnerability. It is one of the characteristics of the secure services that all who form part of it, staff, patients, relatives, are vulnerable but perhaps the patient's position here is overlooked. He, or she, will be seen as the aggressor, the transgressor, who needs containing, 'taming'. That is true but patients, often themselves the victims of abuse early in life, become in detention the responsibility of others and subject to the behaviour and attitudes of both staff and other patients. At one extreme (rare we now hope) there has been overt ill treatment by staff. There were also violent incidents between patients which have resulted in recent years in two murders and several serious injuries. Patients are also vulnerable to their own self-destructive impulses and, despite the staff's vigilance, suicides do occur and self-harm is frequent. A recent study at Rampton Hospital reported 1561 incidents of self-harm by women patients over a 30-month period: an incidence rate of 9.6 per patient per year (Low, Terry and Duggan, in press). It is part of the role of the hospitals to protect patients both from other patients and from themselves: it is a difficult and daunting task.

After discharge or transfer, vulnerability transmutes into stigma. To be an ex-patient from any of the special hospitals carries with it a notoriety and prejudice that make that label a burden which can never be relinquished. It influences the attitudes of professional staff, those in the voluntary sector and makes any reintegration into the community more difficult. Public reaction to the discovery of a neighbour from Broadmoor does not have to be imagined; it has been demonstrated often. As one former patient said:

> I met people in Broadmoor I wouldn't share a house with, but the people from the *News of the World* knock them into a cocked hat. You are terribly penalised if the secret does come out, as happened to me. I lost my whole profession even though I had been out of Broadmoor for 14 years. Once you have that kind of label around your neck, you are completely stigmatised. (*Nursing Times* 1997)

The social indelibility of having been a patient in a special hospital needs to be remembered as one of treatment's incidental legacies.

There are two sizable minorities within the special hospital population who could be seen to be disadvantaged: women and black people. Women patients, although falling in numbers, still account for 15 per cent of current numbers. There is considerable feeling that in the past the culture and setting of a special hospital have been inappropriate and even counter-productive for women with regard to effective treatment (Kaye 1998). This issue is unresolved despite improvements carried out in recent years.

There is considerable evidence that the specific and particular needs of racial minorities within the patient population have not been adequately met. The proportion of this minority is increasing[3] and for the most part is made up of patients of Afro-Caribbean origin although many are now first generation born in England. The black pressure groups vocally condemn the special hospitals as part of a system (including police and prisons) that oppresses the black population; they point to the disproportionately high number of blacks in prison and in the special hospitals (15.2 per cent in special hospitals and 12.67 per cent in prisons as compared to 1.8 per cent in the population at large[4]). There is continuing controversy about diagnosis, treatment and staff attitudes with sufficient evidence to make thoughtful observers uneasy (for instance Bhugra et al. 1996a; 1996b).

A final changing characteristic of the patient population relates to the increasing proportion being admitted from prison[5]. This accelerating influx brings with it particular problems of 'prison culture'. In recent years one of management's aims has been to remove from staff's daily currency those elements and that vocabulary which reflect prisons and their punitive and custodial aims. Paradoxically just those features are being reimported by patients who bring with them expectations and vocabulary which lead them to describe nurses as 'screws' etc. This presents behaviour which the staff can find difficult to overcome, not least an immediate 'them' and 'us' polarity. Whitehall decisions can exacerbate this. On some occasions the Home Office unilaterally transfers a prisoner to a special hospital shortly before his sentence is due to expire. This power is used when the Home Office wants to prevent an individual considered still to be dangerous from re-entering the community. For the special hospitals it means that a patient/prisoner arrives full of resentment at what he will see as further imprisonment, rather than the opportunity for treatment. In our opinion this is a misuse of the Special Hospital facilities.

STAFF

Over the past decade staff have been subject to a pace of change which has been more intensive and more demanding than ever before. In every facet of their social habits they have been expected to relinquish patterns which had long been unchallenged and thus implicitly approved. New requirements have been defined and enthusiastic response demanded. For some this has been water after

---

3   In 1988, 13.4 per cent of admissions to special hospitals were from ethnic minorities compared to 22.9 per cent in 1996.
4   Sources: 1996 ethnic monitoring figures for special hospitals; Home Office Research and Statistics Directorate 1996 for prison population; 1991 Census, Office for National Statistics.
5   In 1988, 23.7 per cent of admissions to special hospitals were from prisons rising to 45.2 per cent in 1996.

the drought, for many a flow to be regarded with some suspicion – 'let's wait and see if it dries up' – and for a significant minority an endangering flood which threatens to sweep away what they have created.

Understandably attention has focused on this last group who have often rallied under the banner of the last of the old-style, reactionary, militant unions – the Prison Officers' Association. That body, representing virtually all categories of staff and at one time the majority of staff, has fought a consistent rearguard action against change, stressing (as it has throughout its history) the overwhelming needs of security to the detriment of therapy. Often it has publicly received a ready welcome for these views – and, occasionally, a sympathetic response from anxious central government figures. Of course on occasion this emphasis has been right: right in the same way that a stopped watch will eventually, if only briefly, be accurate.

In the bewildering mêlée of change and inquiry staff have often been confused and felt like flotsam carried by strong currents towards uncharted destinations. Working in a service where risks and failures have severe and public implications, they have been blamed and punished, individually and collectively (even as this is written a second Ashworth Inquiry is in process with the resignation of the hospital's Chief Executive and a number of staff suspended, awaiting their fate). One does not need much empathy to envisage the effect that this will have on the staff who must continue to persevere in their dangerous, difficult and socially derided task.

The exposure of staff in this fashion is gradually being recognised and steps are being taken to support them both in terms of better preparation, training and clinical supervision and in terms of more consistent support in difficult times. This effort is not yet adequate and there is still a regrettable tendency in any major crisis to regard staff as the most dispensable element in the organisational equation. If any one element will capsize future attempts to reform the service more radically, it will be failure to nurture and support staff. The proper use of directed training which relates closely to practice and practical issues (as for instance in the care of patients with personality disorder) is far from achieved. We continually thrust staff into difficult situations for which they have had little preparation.

Yesterday's isolation which saw them separated from their health service colleagues by virtue of their employment in special hospitals which stood apart is today replaced by the isolation of unfair hazard. Staff are extraordinarily at risk in doing their job and exposed to an unreasonable level of public criticism over their performance. Anxiety about their patients translates to lack of confidence about the staff's judgement and a hasty readiness to vilify and condemn them. The risks are society's risks and the staff – except where their behaviour has been totally unacceptable – must not be punished like the traditional messengers bringing bad news.

'Burn-out' is common among staff although manifestations may vary: some collapse under the strain, others retreat into protective defensive rituals. The new challenges of accepting more responsibility personally and of integrating that into real team-working have, in some cases, proved too much. Many are still struggling with them and others have retreated behind professional barriers as a way of avoiding these difficult issues. The whole basis of professional working has had to be recast: the imperative is on real multidisciplinary teamwork that recognises skills rather than professions and roles rather than hierarchy. This challenges both the dedicated follower ('I do what the doctor says') and the anarchic professional ('we'll do what I say'). In that climate the balance between individual responsibility and the team is not easily found. But if risks are to be minimised and properly understood, the effective team is vital for better treatment of their patients.

MANAGEMENT

The management task was to define a shape and provide a climate: a shape that was recognisable, consistent and realistic; and a climate in which growth could take place safely and fairly. Many of the elements were familiar and had already been described; many of the techniques had already been tested in the wider NHS and in industry. What was unique for the Special Hospitals was bringing all those features together, binding them with a sense of purpose and furthering them with strong resolve. At the time the SHSA was set up, the government gave them the following set of six overall objectives:

- To ensure the continuing safety of the public
- To ensure the provision of appropriate treatment for patients
- To ensure a good quality of life for patients and staff
- To develop the hospitals as centres of excellence for the training of staff in all disciplines in forensic and other branches of psychiatry and psychiatric care and treatment
- To develop closer working relationships with NHS local and regional psychiatric services
- To promote research in fields related to forensic psychiatry.

In philosophical terms the management purpose might be described in terms of Maslow's well-known hierarchy of needs (see Figure 1.2). Along these personal goals can be set the managerial equivalents which the SHSA sought to achieve (see Figure 1.3).[6]

---

6   We are indebted to Dr Dilys Jones, Clinical Strategy Director of the High Security Psychiatric Services Commissioning Board, for allowing us to use this analogy which she originally devised.

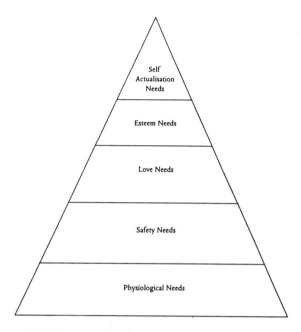

Figure 1.2 Maslow's hierarchy of needs
Source: diagram in *Psychology, the Science of Mind and Behaviour,* Michael D. Gross.

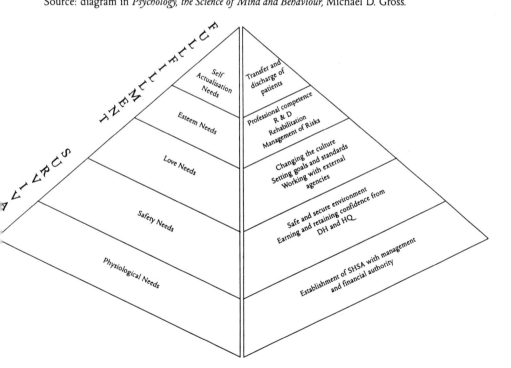

Figure 1.3 Maslow applied to the Special Hospitals
Source: the editors.

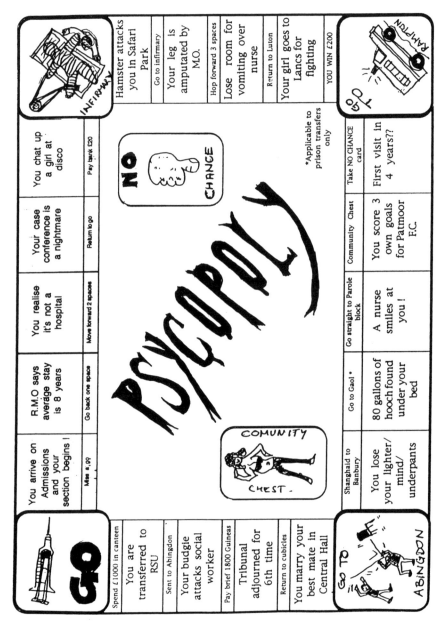

Figure 1.4 'Psychopoly' from the Broadmoor patients' Chronicle

This nice symmetry disguises a volume of difficult practical problems. As with Maslow's original, goals at the base of the hierarchy must be largely achieved before the climb upwards can be undertaken. In this volatile world, the climb can sometimes appear to be a tantalising game of organisational snakes and ladders. Errors and misfortunes in basic areas can and do impede an individual's progress towards the higher levels.

Above all, the demonstration of the safe and secure environment and the creation of a climate of political confidence are the essential prerequisites. That base has to be secured and can never be taken for granted. Damaging incidents will occur – such as the allegations of ill treatment at Ashworth Hospital (1990), the escapes of patients from Broadmoor (1991 and 1992) and Rampton (1994), and allegations of paedophilia at Ashworth Hospital (1997). Each will curtail sharply management's ability to focus on the higher – and more rewarding – levels.

Following chapters describe in detail all aspects of the work to achieve this progression. Some of that work was necessary to overcome setbacks; much of it was delayed by the need to learn and test. Even today it is clear that there is much more to achieve at the top of the hierarchy. Certainly patients move on – many successfully. But we still cannot clearly identify those factors in treatment which contribute directly to such success. The need for more research and greater understanding of the relationship between treatment, illness and recovery remains outstanding. The very variety of patients previously mentioned makes this an enormously complex field – and within the special hospitals are very ill patients, chronic and almost intractable in their illnesses. Even within the hospitals' environments, the process of standard setting and of measuring progress against given standards is still elementary. Too many of the existing measures are clumsily numerical or only 'proxy' evaluations. So, the number of treatment sessions a patient attends is a starting point but only that: how do we progress to the assessment of the effectiveness of particular sessions, or compare the value of one therapy against another? And do that for patients with different illnesses and needs? On a practical level how can we achieve more sophistication in such processes without burdening staff and hospitals with ever increasing paperwork to the detriment of their availability to treat patients directly?

Some of the management effort has had to be on the casting out of the unwanted, a purging both of attitudes and, reluctantly, sometimes of people. That is painful and progress is uneven; you can't wait until everything is perfect before effecting change and we have had to accept imperfections to ensure that the overall impetus did not fade. What is described in the following pages has a unity of purpose and a consistent vision. However its achievement is not complete and progress has not been a straight line. Indeed opinions will vary on the progress made. It is not the end of the story.

REFERENCES

Donovan Report (1997) Paras.4.8 and 12.1. Anglia and Oxford: NHS Executive.

Gross, R.D., (1992) *Psychology, the Science of Mind and Behaviour.* London: Hodder and Stoughton.

HAS (1988) *Health Advisory Service Report on Broadmoor Hospital.* London: HAS.

Home Office (1997) *Home Office Statistical Bulletin.* Issue 20/97, September.

Hutchinson, G., Takei, N., Fahy, T.A. and Bhughra, D. (1996) 'Morbid risk of schizophrenia in first-degree relatives of white and Afro-Caribbean patients with psychosis.' *British Journal of Psychiatry 169*, 6, 776–780.

Kaye, C. (1998) 'Hallmarks of a secure psychiatric service for women.' *Psychiatric Bulletin 22*, 3, March 1998 137–140.

Low, G., Terry, G. and Duggan, C. (1997) 'Deliberate self harm among female patients at a special hospital.' *Health Trends 29*, 1 6–9.

Murphy, E. (1996) 'The past and future of special hospitals.' *Journal of Mental Health 5*, 5, 475–482.

Nature (1996) 27 March, p.310.

Nursing Times, 93, 2, 8 January.

The Mail on Sunday (1997) Editorial, 23 February.

Wood, J. (1995) 'Foreword.' In H. Prins *Offenders, Deviants or Patients?* Second edition. London: Routledge.

CHAPTER 2

Brief History of the Special Hospitals

Charles Kaye

DEVELOPMENT OF THE LAW

In 1800, James Hadfield was found not guilty by reason of insanity of an attempt to kill King George III. Because the court feared that others might be at risk from him in future it ordered his detention in humane conditions. Shortly afterwards in the same year an Act 'for the safe custody of insane persons charged with offences' was passed by Parliament, making statutory provision for the special verdict of not guilty by reason of insanity, and requiring the court to order the detention of the accused, following such a verdict, in strict custody until His Majesty's pleasure was known.

This represents the origins of the present-day concept of the hospital order and restriction order. In Hadfield's case the court's recommendation of mercy and humanity was a reflection of its view that asylum in hospital was more appropriate than imprisonment, and under the 1800 Act it became the Home Secretary's practice to order detention in Bethlem, where a special wing was built in 1815, after a recommendation of a House of Commons' select committee in 1807. By 1848 it had become full and additional provision was made at Fisherton House in Salisbury. This too quickly filled, and in 1856 the Home Secretary took the decision to build a new institution specially for the criminally insane. The Criminal Lunatic Asylums Act 1860 made legal arrangements for the operation of such an asylum.

BROADMOOR HOSPITAL

The site chosen was a plateau in the Berkshire countryside, as the country air was believed to be beneficial to the insane, and the building was designed by a famous architect of the day, Sir Joshua Jebb. The labour was provided by convicts from the Isle of Wight and the buildings were completed within three years.

The first patients to arrive when the institution opened in 1863 were those transferred from local prisons and asylums and Bethlem. These were all 'Her Majesty's Pleasure' patients found not guilty by reason of insanity or insane on arraignment. From 1877 onwards, when prisons came under government control, convicts were admitted. For its first 50 years Broadmoor served the whole of England and Wales.

A regular pattern was quickly established. Persons accused of serious offences, who were found to be insane, were ordered by the Home Secretary to be removed to Broadmoor, as were those who were identified as being insane while serving a term of imprisonment. Patients who were thought no longer to require such secure conditions were transferred to county asylums, and those who were thought to have recovered were discharged, although clearly not as quickly as new patients were admitted. The 500 patients Broadmoor had in the 1860s rose by 1910 to 840, and some mentally disordered prisoners had to be housed in a temporary asylum at Parkhurst on the Isle of Wight.

RAMPTON HOSPITAL

To provide permanent relief from the overcrowding the Home Office built a new institution at Rampton situated in north Nottinghamshire six miles from the nearest town of Retford. It was started in 1908 and opened in 1912 as a northern equivalent of Broadmoor. During the First World War, however, the patient population of the two institutions dropped in numbers. By the end of the war the population of Broadmoor had dropped to a point where the mentally ill patients at Rampton could be moved back, and in 1920 Rampton was taken over by the Board of Control as a secure mental deficiency institution. To help make room for the patients who were brought from Rampton about 100 elderly Broadmoor patients were transferred to county asylums. They were, however, reluctant to accept them and, as Broadmoor continued to have empty beds, they were returned there two years later as a result of pressure from the local asylums.

MOSS SIDE HOSPITAL

In 1904 Liverpool Select Vestry planned to build permanent accommodation for 'the imbecile and epileptic indoor poor of the parish' jointly with the West Derby Union on the Maghull estate on Merseyside, nine miles from Liverpool. However, permission was not given for this to be done. In 1911 Liverpool Select Vestry decided to go ahead on its own with the plans for an epileptic colony, at an estimated cost of £46,500 to accommodate 300 inmates.

The Mental Deficiency Act came into operation on 1 April 1914 and extra accommodation was needed as more patients came under the description of the Act.

In July the incomplete hospital and estate were sold to the Lunacy Board of Control as a State Institution for Defectives for £64,000 but, before it was occupied, they were transferred with the approval of the Home Secretary to the War Office. The hospital was renamed the Military Red Cross Hospital, Moss Side, to be used for the treatment of shell-shocked patients. The first 20 patients were admitted on 7 December 1914. During the war, 3138 patients with shell-shock were admitted to Moss Side Hospital and, even after the armistice, 500 were admitted in the first six months of 1919.

The hospital was handed back to the Lunacy Board in August 1919 and a few patients from Parkhurst prison were temporarily accepted. The hospital was used by the Ministry of Pensions for the treatment of patients until October 1933 when Rampton was full and Moss Side Hospital, which had 256 beds, took 100 patients from Rampton. Patients continued to be transferred from Rampton and in 1938 the hospital had 239 patients. Additional accommodation was built on the east site in the 1940s and by 1945 the hospital had 375 inpatients.

In 1990 Moss Side was formally amalgamated with the adjacent Park Lane Hospital to form Ashworth Hospital. In the process of reorganisation, the original Moss Side buildings were closed in 1995.

PARK LANE HOSPITAL

By the 1970s, a fourth special hospital was needed to relieve chronic overcrowding at Broadmoor. The original Harrison estate still had a large area of farming land to the north of Moss Side Hospital which was a suitable site and 50 acres of land were released to build the new Park Lane Special Hospital.

In 1974, Park Lane Hospital was opened on a temporary basis in two former Moss Side wards with the administration offices in portakabins. Two years later, major building work started on the permanent hospital, which was completed in 1984, although groups of completed wards were gradually commissioned during this period.

MANAGEMENT

Direct Home Office management of Broadmoor ceased with the Criminal Justice Act 1948, when the term 'criminal lunatic' was abolished and the hospital management passed to the Board of Control. However, it remained solely for the use of mentally ill offenders, and admissions as well as discharges were the sole responsibility of the Home Secretary. It was not until the new legal arrangements established by the Mental Health Act 1959 and the Emery Report (Ministry of Health 1961) on the special hospitals, that the way was opened for the admission of patients under civil as well as criminal powers of detention.

Key differences between Broadmoor on the one hand and Moss Side and Rampton on the other were that the former took no mental defectives, and similarly only took offenders who had been before a court. The latter two institutions found themselves admitting both offenders and non-offenders. Broadmoor was run by the Home Office until April 1949 when it was taken over by the Ministry of Health and run by the Board of Control, in accordance with changes of the Criminal Justice Act 1948. Admissions and discharges continued to be regulated by the Home Office. Rampton and Moss Side, when caring for mental defectives, were run by the Board of Control. Management by the Board continued even when ownership was transferred to the Ministry of Health with the advent of the 1946 National Health Service Act.

The 1959 Mental Health Act renamed the three institutions, defined their purpose and altered their admissions policies. Broadmoor, Moss Side and Rampton became 'Special Hospitals'. They were the designated hospitals for individuals later deemed to be in need of 'treatment under conditions of special security on account of their dangerous, violent or criminal propensities' (NHS Act 1977). They were able to admit anyone who fell under one of the categories of the 1959 Mental Health Act – mental illness, subnormality, severe subnormality or psychopathic disorder – whether or not they had been charged to appear in the criminal court. This arrangement was confirmed by the 1983 Mental Health Act.

Until 1989 the hospitals were administered directly by the Ministry of Health, later the Department of Health and Social Security. In that year a new health authority (the Special Hospitals Service Authority – SHSA) was formed to manage the hospitals and their service. This brought the hospitals in line with the prevailing management culture and arrangements within the NHS and saw, importantly, the introduction of the concept of general management into the hospitals.

The SHSA was never envisaged as a permanent arrangement – its initial charter allowed for a review after three years – and following interdepartmental deliberations it was decided that it should be dissolved. Accordingly in 1996 each special hospital was created an Authority in its own right (similar to an NHS Trust) and a new purchasing body – the High Security Psychiatric Services Commissioning Board – was created as part of the NHS Executive.

CHAPTER 3

Autobiographies

Charles Kaye: The Story of his Involvement

In the summer of 1989 I was district general manager of the Health Authority at Basingstoke in Hampshire and had worked in that district in a variety of roles since the late 1970s but was very much in the mood for change. I was aware that the same problems were returning for further review and that a long history of working in the district, and often taking unpopular decisions, was to a significant extent getting in the way of progress. I was also extremely disappointed that there had been no enthusiasm either from the Health Authority itself or from the units in the Authority for the creation of first wave Trusts. I had made a proposal for two such Trusts to be put forward and had received very little support from any quarter. I was quite clear that it was time to move on.

However, the problem was where to move and what to do. I could see little benefit in going to another health district and doing the same sort of job as I had been doing for the last four years or so. A larger district, different problems superficially, but it seemed to me to have the feeling just of going back and of not doing something new. So I was on the look-out for jobs that had a flavour of something different, that were health service linked, but not necessarily in the conventional district orientation. I had applied for a regional manager's job and reached the last two but such jobs were limited and I couldn't afford to wait indefinitely for more to come up. In this mood I had looked at one or two of the new agencies that were being created in line with the Whitehall changes, and I saw advertised the post of Chief Executive to the Special Hospitals Service Authority which was just about to come into being. My first-hand knowledge of the special hospitals was non-existent although, coincidentally, I had just signed an education agreement with them with regard to the training of student nurses at our school in Basingstoke. As far as their work and role were concerned I knew no more than the man in the street and, of course, his knowledge, as now, is prejudice and stereotype rather than real awareness.

However, the prospect intrigued me and it certainly fitted my requirements in terms of being health-connected but not a health district in the conventional sense. I applied and began to make enquiries and contacts to see what the job consisted of. One of these contacts was Cliff Graham, the key civil servant at the Department of Health, whom I discovered was the architect of the creation of the SHSA. As soon as I mentioned an interest to him he enthusiastically responded and came to see me at Basingstoke to talk about the job. What he described sounded both daunting and exciting. For the first time I heard about the role and power of the Prison Officers' Association (POA) and the curious and unexpected role played by Jimmy Savile at Broadmoor Hospital. I visited Broadmoor Hospital and was shown round by Moyra Rogue. As I had no idea what to expect I am not sure if I was surprised but I certainly responded with some very strong impressions. Firstly, there was the wall. As you came up the drive and climbed towards the hospital and turned a corner there in front of you was the wall. Solid, rising, red with black detail and signifying one of the key essentials of Broadmoor Hospital. On the tour around the hospital, which of course starts in the new accommodation in the administration block, we quickly went to Norfolk House which was then the site for the male intensive care ward. At that time you walked down into the ward on the ground floor and it really felt like descending into a pit. The fabric was grim, institutional and neglected, and the atmosphere was tense and antagonistic, conveying strongly much of what I later came to identify as the negative inheritance of the SHSA. However, none of that actually succeeded in putting me off and shortly afterwards I turned up for interview at the Grafton Hotel in Tottenham Court Road.

The very short-list was an indication of moving in a different world. Besides myself there was a consultant psychiatrist working in a regional secure unit, an ex-prison governor, now a member of the Inspector of Prisons' staff, and two health general managers, both of whom I knew and one of whom used to work for me. In that curious, superstitious way that still influences us, I noted that the interviews were taking place in the Fitzroy Suite which I took to be a good omen (that being one of my Christian names), and after a battery of psychometric testing and a formal interview I got the job. I had been very impressed with the chairman, David Edmond, and was keen to get on with the work. There was the usual gap of nearly three months between July when I was appointed and 23 October when I started, but that period was far from inactive so far as I and the SHSA were concerned. Firstly, there was the question of the appointment of general managers for the three hospitals. David and I discussed this and I accepted his judgement that the appointment of the incumbent medical director at Rampton Hospital, Diana Dickens, was the right way to go forward. An interviewing panel was set up for Broadmoor Hospital where Alan Franey, the administrator with a task-force was appointed, at a time when I was away and couldn't attend. At those interviews another candidate apparently sank his chances by talking about standing on a tank and addressing his troops! That left Park Lane and Moss Side Hospitals where advertisement had failed to attract the right candidates. I asked Brian Johnson, the incumbent chief nursing officer at Park Lane, to come and see me and I talked to him about the job and David and I agreed that he should be appointed. During my absence on holiday I also discovered, with a certain amount of disappointment, that David and Cliff Graham had gone ahead and appointed one of the unsuccessful candidates for my job as one of my directors! This move, however well-intentioned, created tensions and ambiguities which took a long time and a lot of effort to resolve.

Thus, in October when I arrived at Charles House, which would be our 'temporary offices', I had a director whom I hadn't personally appointed and a handful of staff transferred from the Department of Health, in fact those individuals who had been concerned in the running of the special hospitals from the Department. I also received a long list from the Department of the issues that they thought should be addressed.

I needed to set up a headquarters staff which would give the right messages and the right leadership to the hospitals. I had also to talk positively and convincingly to the outside world. I had enormous tasks, the full dimensions of which I didn't really appreciate, and the need to become acquainted with the three hospitals. I had to lead my general managers towards changes and improvements which had to be achieved – and speedily. Little time for reflection. I also found myself operating at a political level with the Department of Health and the Home Office that was new to me – although not unattractive. At the same time we were drawing together a new Authority (one of the first to be put together on the executive and non-executive principles) whose members were themselves strangers to each other.

I had already two important allies; the post of director of medical services had been advertised and received significant attention, and I had been visited by two Doctors Taylor in my fastness at Basingstoke. One of these was Pamela Taylor whom we were happy to appoint as director and who, in terms of credibility, intellectual ability and clinical acumen, was extremely successful. We had also interviewed for the post of director of nursing services and had appointed Frank Powell who came with excellent background and credentials.

Thus, I started in earnest on 23 October 1989 with the assets of some important individuals appointed, although only one had taken up her post; with some knowledgeable civil servants, not all of whom were sure that they wanted to work for a health authority; with a fair amount of guidance from the Department's civil servants; with a number of warnings regarding what was expected of the new Authority; and an awareness that my health service principles would need to be maintained. My skills as a general manager in shaping policies and leading others towards them were about to be put to the biggest test that I had experienced. I knew that there would be a challenge or perhaps a series of challenges from the POA. I knew there would be scepticism from the staff and from the world outside about whether the SHSA could achieve anything. This sceptical, not to say hostile, attitude was summed up by an early event when David and I met the Chairman and Vice-Chairman of the Mental Health Act Commission, Louis Blom-Cooper and Elaine Murphy, for a private dinner in Soho. Before we'd even sat down for the meal Louis Blom-Cooper had announced in his typical jocular style that the only thing you could do with the Special Hospitals was burn them to the ground. As their newly appointed Chief Executive I was determined and certain that you could improve them, that you could bring the right values and the right goals to each hospital and that we would demonstrate that the Blom-Cooper anarchic solution was not only impracticable but also unnecessary.

I had met two of the general managers; Alan Franey was obviously tough and determined, Brian Johnson knowledgeable and enthusiastic. At that stage, although I knew I'd look for a close working relationship with them, I had no way of predicting how that would turn out. Diana Dickens proved to be somebody who was harder to get to know and more difficult to find the right relationship with. But the essentials of the team were now present and it was up to me to lead them towards change.

What was the attraction? First, this post was certainly as different as I had mused on back in the summer in Hampshire. Second, it offered plenty of challenges and difficulties, many of them in different areas from those that I'd dealt with previously and I was ready for those sorts of challenges.

Third, it was an organisation which needed to be shaped from the start which I know from my previous experience was a situation that attracted me. I have always been far more interested in taking over something new and giving it a shape than in inheriting something and continuing it in a previously determined mode. Fourth, and perhaps in some ways the most significant point, I could see that the patients and, in a curious way, the staff were disadvantaged and indeed despised in many respects by the rest of the world. It seemed to me worth trying to change those attitudes, giving the staff self-respect in doing a difficult and exacting job, and trying to give patients better opportunities for the future. Thus started seven years' hard work.

Alan Franey: The Story of his Involvement

In 1987 working as Deputy Secretary at the National Institute of Biological Standards and Control I was approached by the Senior Department of Health Civil Servant and asked whether I would consider a secondment for a six-week period to Broadmoor Hospital as part of a task-force. Having spent my entire career in the NHS working at hospitals in Brighton, London and Leeds I found the thought of working within Broadmoor somewhat daunting, never having thought of it previously. I had an unusual meeting in the Athenaeum Club in London with some officials who shall remain nameless and I was persuaded that a move to Broadmoor Hospital would be a good career step.

In October 1988 I arrived on the back of a very highly critical Health Advisory Service report which described the hospital as 'an inward looking institution with some very doubtful methods of dealing with disturbed behaviour', and the message was clear: 'change it or close it'. There were over 200 recommendations; I had the daunting task of drawing up an action plan and the then Minister, Edwina Currie, thought that could be achieved in six weeks. It was some six months later that I discovered that the then government intended to set up the Special Hospitals Service Authority, and introduce into the three special hospitals general management which had been in place in the NHS since the early 1980s. I applied for the post, was successful and started my role as general manager at Broadmoor Hospital in the summer of 1989. The following years were to be very challenging both for me and for the hospital itself as I was determined to lead a team that would bring about real change and that meant, for everyone concerned, a rethink about what they were doing within the organisation. It was a major learning curve for me and I remember in the early days turning up at 6 a.m. and spending the day on the wards talking to patients and staff and finding out for myself some of the pressures that the carers were facing. I met many staff who had been working at the hospital for a good number of years and had a very custodial approach towards their work. They tended to look at patients as criminals who had committed horrendous crimes rather than individuals with a mental disorder that required treatment. Later in this book you will read about some of the issues that had to be tackled not only at Broadmoor Hospital but at Ashworth and Rampton Hospitals as well and I hope that by the time you have come to the end of the book you will see evidence of a shift in culture and real change in the way special hospitals have been managed in recent years.

REFERENCES

HAS (1988) *Health Advisory Service Report on Broadmoor Hospital.* London: HAS.

PART 2

Challenging the Institution

CHAPTER 4

The Inheritance
Charles Kaye and Alan Franey

I was locked up in Broadmoor, the most institutional of institutions, for almost nine years. As a patient, you live, eat and sleep the place, and it is not much different for the staff. But the staff uniforms and the fact that they were members of the Prison Officers' Association (POA) emphasised the divide between staff and patients. (Allen 1997)

Perhaps the most relevant image of the Special Hospitals in the mid 1980s is that of isolated islands: off-shore both to the health service (which would see them as prisons) and to the criminal justice system (which would regard them as settings for care in custody). While having links and allegiances to both government departments, and trying to please both in their operation, the special hospitals remained distant, separated from the assurance of the mainland by a turbid channel which made them both inaccessible and vulnerable.

That isolation had a number of manifestations and consequences which together formed the deposit that the SHSA took over in 1989. The four hospitals (Park Lane and Moss Side, although adjacent, were quite separate as institutions) clearly shared at that time the conflict of role – between 'therapy' and 'security'. There was confusion internally resulting both from poorly focused administrative arrangements, and from the absence of any wider strategic direction. To its credit the Department of Health clearly saw the need for change to remedy those defects. In particular Cliff Graham, then Under Secretary, was instrumental in creating a climate which allowed the introduction of a new organisation to manage, correct and revitalise the three sites. The Department of Health summarised the tasks facing the SHSA in two admirable documents in 1989 (Department of Health 1989a; 1989b) but their careful prose, which mapped out what should be, only fleetingly touched on the inadequacy (despite the best efforts of many devoted staff) of what existed.

It would be quite wrong to assume that every aspect of each of the hospitals was at that time negative and anti-therapeutic. There were welcome examples of individual professionals and services outstanding in their aims and achievements. But more often than not skilled staff were frustrated by the overall negativity, indifference or outright opposition of their colleagues and superiors. The prevailing values were custodial: at best paternal, at worst punitive. Above all the impetus, encouragement and permission to think and act therapeutically were missing: this was one of the principal gaps that the SHSA and its managers sought to fill.

Any account of the hospitals' everyday life at that time is going to be impressionistic but the flavour of those impressions is important. The following snapshots concentrate on six aspects: staff and attitudes, environment and atmosphere, language, administration, the outside world and patients' lives.

STAFF AND ATTITUDES

Virtually all the staff were members of the Prison Officers' Association. This union is based principally in prisons, originally founded in Wormwood Scrubs in 1938 and established in Broadmoor in 1949. As Professor Thomas says in his authoritative study:

> ...it is necessary to note its contribution to every increase in public concern, through its constant allegations of defects at Annual Conferences, in its magazine and elsewhere. (Thomas 1972)

This overwhelming emphasis on security – as would be expected from a warders' union – was imported unadulterated into the special hospitals. If to this allegiance is added the standard dress[1] of the nurses – prison officers' uniforms, peaked caps and Doc Marten boots – the stage is set. The predominant approach of the nursing staff was custodial; warders first, nurses second, with the keys and the uniforms the great symbols of authority and control. To watch shifts change at Broadmoor and see the nurses emerge with peaked caps, military style, was to realise the urgent need for change.

The POA were strong because they were effective. They defended their members vigorously and at a time when those members had virtually no support from any other source. As a union, in the short term, they delivered; but simultaneously and almost inevitably they transmitted through their organisation the prevailing values of the prisons: detention, restraint, toughness, a 'macho' culture where the biggest and most violent patient (or prisoner) would be brought into submission. Nurses accordingly developed a carapace beneath which they could survive (even if at the expense of their professional

---

1   Park Lane Hospital was an exception since its nurses had not worn uniform since it opened in 1974.

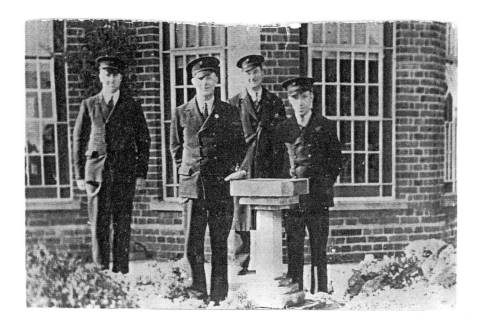

Figure 4.1 Rampton Hospital staff in the 1940s

values). Such attitudes were shared by members of other professions working in the hospitals.

The pervasiveness of these attitudes was heavily reinforced by the staff estates which provided something close to a *cordon sanitaire* around the hospitals, sealing them off from their surroundings. Large numbers of staff, and not only nurses, lived in the hospital houses, with other staff as neighbours, and used the hospital social club and sporting facilities as a principal source of recreation and leisure. Whole families, spread over generations, could work at the hospital with connections by marriage reinforcing the bonds. In 1992 an enrolled nurse retired who had worked in Broadmoor Hospital (apart from war service) since he joined it as a 14-year-old 'doctor's boy' in 1940. He was the third generation of his family to work in the hospital and when his son joined the staff in the mid 1970s – making it four generations – there were 13 relatives of his working in the hospital. Add the informal networks and connections in such communities and you begin to appreciate the sheer pressure to conform to the prevailing pattern of behaviour.

These social bonds were subtly reinforced by the financial rewards attached to Special Hospital work. Paradoxically the very recognition of the exacting nature of the work – and the attendant dangers – encouraged the Department of Health to introduce an additional premium (the Special Hospital lead) which, coupled with a generous approach to grading to aid recruitment, created golden chains which bound many staff to their jobs. Given relatively high pay, a hospital house, family connections and a tradition of local service, many staff stayed in the hospitals for years, even a whole lifetime. There was a nationally negotiated 'promotion' policy which meant that service in each grade was required before promotion, providing official endorsement of progress by seniority, rather than by ability. The inward-looking, traditional and conservative viewpoints were thus reinforced and 'outsiders' seeking change in the middle of the organisation were effectively muffled and marginalised, either eventually accepting the norm or moving on in frustration (often accompanied by a personal bitterness). The prevailing view was that you had to serve your time to entitle you to 'join the club'.

Relationships between the bulk of the staff, the nurses, and the other trained staff were uneasy. While the key role of the doctors was acknowledged, there existed an unwritten agreement between doctors and nurses about professional boundaries, leaving the nurses in exclusive charge of the day-to-day management of patients. Other professionals, psychologists and social workers for example, were often resented and characterised as 'interfering' and being 'soft'. At Broadmoor in 1988 they were discouraged from going onto the wards after 5p.m. unless they requested, and were granted by the charge nurse, specific permission for such a visit. Indeed the senior managers were expected to make an appointment to visit a ward.

Predominantly it was a male culture with women staff very much a minority. It was rare to see in any of the hospitals male and female nurses working on the same ward; male nurses were on the men's wards and females on the women's wards. The specific effects of that on women patients are detailed elsewhere but overall this male domination added a certain harshness to regimes and behaviour.

ENVIRONMENT AND ATMOSPHERE

Although there had been a substantial capital investment, certainly since the building of Park Lane Hospital, the physical environment was bleak and discouraging. Park Lane had new buildings but they were set in a featureless 'moonscape' raked by harsh winds and with no attempt to soften the stark brickwork of the building or the impact of the full prison standard boundary wall with projecting 'beak'. Even there two wards were still not in use nearly a decade after the first buildings on site were commissioned.

Broadmoor had indeed a new wing, delayed and constructed considerably over budget, but not occupied because of staff objections to new systems and 'security risks'. The best wards in the hospital were empty because the staff would not use them. Most of the remaining buildings in the hospital, built in the mid 1860s, were overcrowded with a number of large dormitories which were almost 'no-go' areas to staff at night. Conditions in Norfolk House, housing the intensive care unit for the most disturbed patients, were particularly bad.

In Moss Side, the external environment was attractive in the style of many large psychiatric hospitals, with pleasant gardens and a large pond. The wards, however, set in such surroundings were severely institutional, reflecting and engendering the unacceptable procedures identified so graphically in the public inquiry into allegations of abuse at Ashworth Hospital published in 1992. All the wards had been adapted for high security psychiatric care and presented major problems with regard to overcrowding, observation of patients and inadequate supporting accommodation (interview rooms, occupational therapy and recreational space).

> Ashworth South wards were unacceptably bare and unwelcoming and were pervaded by an atmosphere of hopeless inactivity. (Ashworth Report 1992)

Communication between the two Merseyside hospitals was limited to such an extent that it was difficult to believe they were side by side on the same campus. They had different security and key systems so that staff could not pass freely between them and very little interchange of staff or patients took place, thus denying Moss Side residents the opportunity to use the much superior workshop and recreational facilities at Park Lane. In many instances there was downright hostility between the staff of the two hospitals. Many of the Moss Side staff felt the regime at Park Lane was 'soft'.

Rampton was a mixture with an inner core of wards in three-storey oppressive buildings urgently in need of renovation (work had started on one of these blocks). These were linked by a corridor system whose décor would silence the most optimistic and light-hearted. None of the lessons learned elsewhere about the treatment of such areas with colour and design had reached north Nottinghamshire. An outer ring of villas were more congenial, set in pleasant surroundings. But again internally they were inadequate and urgently in need of bringing up to modern hospital standards.

The first phase of major redevelopment had started but was of infrastructure, boiler house etc. Throughout the hospitals there was uneven provision of basic facilities for patients: heating, call systems, personal storage, single rooms, facilities for exercise inside and outside the wards.

Interestingly, in the very area of physical security, standards were uneven. Park Lane was fully surrounded by the wall described above while Moss Side had no more than a simple wire fence. Both the other hospitals had serious gaps in their perimeter security precautions. The varying standards of external security had the effect of reinforcing the staff's custodial approach to care. Weaknesses in the physical security encouraged staff to focus on control. If more liberal regimes were to be practised internally, these defects would have to be remedied to avoid compromising overall security.

LANGUAGE

Often unconsciously what is spoken is the barometer of feelings more deeply held – and perhaps concealed. As Gaston Bacheland, quoted by Murray Cox, puts it: 'But the image has touched the depths before it stirs the surface.' (Cox and Theilgaard 1987, p.xiii)

Expressions familiar in prisons were (and to some extent still are) used regularly in the hospitals. Thus:

- o 'occupations' instead of diversional and occupational therapy
- o 'airing courts' for courtyards or gardens where patients could walk
- o 'association' for patients meeting each other
- o 'parole' for patients allowed greater freedom of movement within the hospital
- o 'nonce' for sexual offender
- o 'gallery' for corridor
- o 'slopping out' for emptying chamber pots
- o 'mess room' for staff room
- o 'scullery' for kitchen
- o 'locking off' for restricting access to corridors
- o 'grass' for informer.

It was said to be common for patients to refer to others as 'wops', 'low grades', 'mess pots', phrases picked up from staff. (Ashworth Report 1992)

On the Merseyside campus there was a small but active group of National Front sympathisers who regularly circulated offensive material and issued threats to staff who they felt did not share their way of looking at the hospital. There were known National Front sympathisers in Broadmoor as well.

ADMINISTRATION

The pre-SHSA situation has been delicately described as 'the uncertain distribution of managerial powers' (Ashworth Report 1992).

What existed was a troika arrangement which had already been discarded in the mainstream NHS in favour of general management and a clear allocation of responsibility for decision making.

In 1988 each hospital had a management team consisting of the Medical Director, Chief Nursing Officer and Administrator. Park Lane and Moss Side shared the same Administrator. None of the three had any managerial authority over the others although in practice the Medical Director could appear to be '*primus inter pares*'. These teams were responsible both to the Department of Health (in the shape of the Special Hospital Service Board, a body of multiprofessional civil servants chaired by an Under Secretary) and to their local hospital boards, an assembly of lay persons, who themselves had delegated responsibilities from the Department, mainly in respect of complaints, statutory mental health manager duties and, theoretically, the determination of priorities and the development of resources

Given such a complicated structure, given the organisational proximity of the civil servants in the Department and the political sensitivities always attendant on the special hospitals, it is not surprising that clear policy making and decision taking were strangers to these management bodies. A paralysis of pressures rendered the most determined players impotent and afforded ample excuse for the faint-hearted to evade the difficult and unpleasant. Interprofessional conflicts and tribalism could flourish and interference was the order of the day. As the Health Advisory Service described it at Broadmoor:

> In practice many functions are retained by the DHSS and the interventionist actions of its officers are often confusing, misunderstood and sometimes resented. Board members, members of the HMT and hospital staff generally are uncertain about management roles and responsibilities. Delineation of managerial work and authority between the various tiers and teams is unclear. Credible leadership is not obvious. Organisational philosophy and style are not shared. Most management activity is conducted at too high a level. Decision taking on policy issues is slow and cumbersome because excessive detail and trivia are dealt with by the most senior officers. Incoherent management change and uncertainty in the immediate past have been detrimental to morale development and sound management practices. (NHS and DHSS 1988, pp.22–23)

Civil servants could see the need to set policy and make it happen operationally but were not in a position to do so themselves. Conversely others in the management merry-go-round were inhibited by lack of clarity about their own responsibilities and by restraints imposed by other layers. Check and balance brought matters virtually to a halt and allowed the POA to move into a managerial vacuum and make the running. This was illustrated in 1987 industrial action at Moss Side when local management's stand against the POA was, in their eyes, undercut by the Department's reversal of a key decision. The civil servants were understandably nervous about tackling such difficult issues and this hesitation at national level strengthened the POA's hold locally.

RELATIONSHIPS WITH THE WORLD OUTSIDE

The hospitals had always to deal with the duality of being managed by the Department of Health while being subject to the authority of the Home Office in terms of decisions about the future of individual restricted patients. Having to satisfy the requirements of the two Departments created its own tensions. Although many of the doctors related well to the officials in the Home Office there was widespread feeling that their procedures caused delays in the movement of patients. The Home Office always made clear its role: the overriding concern of the Home Office is the protection of the public (Home Office 1989, p.5). It was supportive of the managerial changes provided that it would have the opportunity to monitor the SHSA's work, both through its nominated non-executive members on the Authority and through regular contact with the SHSA Executive and the Department of Health. To the Home Office, the Special Hospitals were an essential resource.

More widely, attitudes towards the hospitals were rather less positive. Pressure groups in the fields of mental health and prison reform saw them as at best, ineffective, and at worst, brutalising.

> Whatever the answer the SHSA comes up with, one thing is clear: there is a good case for closing the special hospitals. Long associated with scandal and patient abuse, squalor and isolation, they stand as a monument to a different age. They cannot be rehabilitated. (Ros Hepplewhite, National Director of MIND (Openmind 1990/1991))

At an early meeting with Sir Louis Blom-Cooper, Chairman designate of the Mental Health Act Commission, the newly appointed Chief Executive of the SHSA was told that the only thing to do with the hospitals was to burn them to the ground.

Conversely, within the NHS, the hospitals were seen as rather privileged places, being well supplied with staff and resources, protected from NHS 'cuts' and yet still not providing a reliable service, often delaying admission of violent and difficult patients.

PATIENTS AND REGIMES

In the lives of patients the key notes were restriction and routine:

> ...Broadmoor was a place of discipline not only for the patients but for the staff as well. (Charles Lynch, Nurse 1964–96, Broadmoor Hospital (in *Broadly Speaking* interview, 1996))

In typically institutional fashion the business of the ward would be arranged inflexibly and become a programme into which each patient was to fit. Learning how to adopt (and sometimes with experience adapt) the routine was a necessary survival skill for the patient. By the same token, such conforming behaviour was seen by staff as a key indicator of a patient's progress. As one consultant described the scene:

> We have endured a repressive, intimidating anti-therapeutic culture over the years. At times work at Ashworth Hospital has been turgid, frightening, even monotonous. This is the view of a member of staff talking. What of the patients? Serially invalidated over the years themselves gradually losing more and more of their individuality and their capacity to survive. I do not talk of all patients, nor of all staff. Some patients have 'nous' and do survive; some do fight, albeit feebly. (Dr Peter Gravett, quoted in HMSO (1992))

Even at Park Lane, the newest of the hospitals, there was a regular daily practice of herding the patients in an escorted crocodile between the wards and their workshops. Four times a day this demeaning procession trouped across the site. A senior nurse recounts how in 1988 at Park Lane, staff on one ward took some patients outside their ward to kick a football around. Nurses in an adjacent ward phoned the Chief Nursing Officer to complain about this 'luxury' being offered to patients.

A typical day in a ward at Broadmoor in the late 1980s would follow this pattern:

Day in the life of a patient

7.00	Woken up
7.10	Shaving time – given razor under supervision
7.45	Breakfast
8.15	Medication
9.00	Occupations
12.00	Lunch
13.30	Occupations / Education
17.00	Tea
20.00	Medication
20.45	Lock-up

Patients would dress and undress in the corridors of the wards, outside their rooms, in the full and public view of the ward staff and any other visitors – privacy was not considered appropriate; indeed it would be regarded as breaching security. At Rampton, patients were compelled to leave their shoes outside their rooms at night, allegedly to demonstrate that they were in their rooms.

When patients made their beds they were expected to do this in military style with blankets and sheets folded in a particular fashion.

At breaks in the morning and afternoon when tea was served for the patients, it would be made in one very large teapot with the milk added to the pot since separate jugs for milk would be considered potential weapons and a security risk.

Patients would be viewed in terms of their offence and its perceived severity, of social unacceptability, rather than in terms of their illness. Conversely some patients would be adopted as ward 'pets' and enjoyed a favoured status.

If you knew what he'd done, you wouldn't sit next to him. (Broadmoor nurse to visiting professional, 1989)

Clinical practices in some instances were dubious: seclusion was regularly used as punishment for 'bad' behaviour. An unwritten guideline, often observed, was that if a patient assaulted a member of staff which resulted in that individual taking sick leave, the patient would be secluded for the period of the sick leave.

As part of the techniques of controlling and restraining patients, staff were taught that it was useful to hit a patient across the knuckles with a bunch of keys that every staff member carried. This was a way of issuing a warning and, of course, of reinforcing physical domination.

All patients were literally locked up all night and would only be visited in an emergency; the majority of rooms did not even have a call system to allow a patient to contact a nurse. Most wards had only one nurse (often unqualified) on duty at night. Additional nurses would have to be summoned from elsewhere if a room was to be entered. Most patients had to urinate and defecate into a pot in their room which stood overnight and had to be emptied by the patient the next morning in a 'slopping out' routine.

Wards were cramped and overcrowded:

This overcrowding meant of course that some wards would be seething. (Charles Lynch, Nurse 1964–96, Broadmoor Hospital)

Norfolk House at Broadmoor provided on the ground floor the hospital's intensive care unit for the most disturbed and disruptive patients. The physical conditions in 1988 were appalling with totally inadequate facilities and standards of decoration that would make 'institutional' a term of praise. The ward was dominated by the 'fear factor' which applied to both staff and patients. With 12 patients resident, the system employed was that six would be allowed out of their rooms whilst the remainder were locked up. At intervals the two groups would exchange locations, irrespective of specific therapeutic needs. The prevailing atmosphere was of continual noise and tension threatening the control by staff.

Patients' sexuality and sexual activity was officially denied and unofficially condoned – within certain limits. Sexual contact, either of a heterosexual or homosexual nature, was not formally allowed. However on one ward in Moss Side the lavatories were separated into two sections: one for the 'queers' and one for the remaining patients. Some degree of physical contact was acknowledged and dealt with by a 'blind eye' approach. This was the trained nursing staff's conventional approach to patients for many of whom sexual abuse or aberrant sexual behaviour was a major factor in their illness or offending.

SUMMARY

It is all too easy to be incredulous and scornful about the picture that such descriptions draw. Such patterns existed because they had been allowed by management to develop, because those responsible at all levels had not found ways of working together to ensure that right values and good practice – both well-defined – prevailed. Although those members of staff who erred were often depicted as sadists and bullies, in a very real sense they were as much victims as the patients they abused. Professor J. P. Martin has tellingly described this as 'the corruption of care':

> By this is meant the fact that primary aims of care – the cure or alleviation of suffering – have become subordinate to what are essentially secondary aims such as the creation and preservation of order, quiet and cleanliness. (Martin 1984)

If to this is added the deep ambivalence in society towards the population of the special hospitals and the acts those individuals committed (often shared by staff who are members of that society) it is possible to understand and to explain this process of erosion – but not to condone it.

By the same token those who would cleanse the stables with thunderbolts of righteous indignation were equally unhelpful. Utopian indulgences would not bring about change: deep-rooted attitudes and practices were established realities, thriving on neglect and indifference. Illuminating them was a start but it would not magically frighten them away. In a very real sense the country had the special hospitals it had helped to create. Those professions which claimed the skills and techniques to curb, modify and even change the behaviour of mentally ill patients would first have to focus on the task of redirecting their colleagues towards behaviour and goals which were therapeutically reasoned and caringly applied.

REFERENCES

Allen, C. (1997) *Nursing Times*. 26 March.

Ashworth Report (1992) *Report of the Committee of Inquiry into Complaints about Ashworth Hospital*. Vol.1, p.146.

Cox, M. and Theilgaard, A. (1987) *Mutative Metaphors in Psychotherapy*. London: Jessica Kingsley Publishers.

Department of Health (1989a) *Operational Brief (May)*. London: DH.

Department of Health (1989b) *Policy Guidelines (October)*. London: DH.

HMSO (1992) *Report of the Committee of Inquiry into Complaints about Ashworth Hospital*. London: HMSO.

Home Office (1989) *Mentally Disordered Offenders*. London: HMSO.

Martin, J.P. (1984) *Hospitals in Trouble*. Oxford: Basil Blackwell Publishers.

NHS and DHSS (1988) *Report on the Services Provided by Broadmoor Hospital*. London: NHS, HAS and DHSS SSI.

Openmind (1990/1991) No.48 (Dec 1990/Jan 1991) p.30.

Thomas, J.E. (1972) *The English Prison Officer since 1850*. London: Routledge and Kegan Paul.

CHAPTER 5

Changing the Spots

Tackling the Culture

Charles Kaye and Alan Franey

Those giant special hospitals, those monuments to nineteenth century tradition and prejudice should surely be regarded as obsolete... (Paul Mullen 1996)

INTRODUCTION

Any commitment to working in or with the special hospitals involves a taxing balancing act between the expedient and the Utopian, between amelioration and abolition. Clearly, like the Irishman's directions, most of us would not have wanted to start from the position evident in the late 1980s. The faults, failures and frustration pent up within the system presented a discouraging catalogue which it would have been easy to read and write off as a hopeless case beyond reform. Indeed the hospitals provided a professional graveyard for many would-be reformers. This understandable reaction was nicely encapsulated during the course of an interview which the Chief Executive had a year after his appointment. The interviewer was Dave Pilgrim working on behalf of MIND; he had previously and unhappily been Principal Clinical Psychologist at Moss Side Hospital (1983–86). He summed up the interview as follows:

> After the interview I was left with uneasy feelings. Is it possible to believe that the hopeful and intelligent attitudes demonstrated by the Chief Executive of the SHSA will really translate into practice? My impression was of a man who in one sense was highly sophisticated in his account of a new-broom policy, but in another sense he was naïvely optimistic.

> At the end of it all, nothing he said convinced me that there should be a place for large, maximum security hospitals in a civilized society. As for the

policy of openness, that is of course to be welcomed. All it may do, though, is reveal more problems to a previously ignorant outside world.

My hunch is that scandals will keep recurring in the special hospital system, and so the sooner that steps are taken to close it down, the better. (Pilgrim 1990/1991)

Pessimism sired by failure out of inertia was a vigorous runner!

We considered that we were in a significantly different position from any previous reformers for three principal reasons:

1.   We were starting at the top with a new team, health service-trained and oriented, untainted by previous compromise or scandal.

2.   We acted in a fluid context where change was expected and innovation possible. The national current would help us, both in terms of the ethos and practice of general management in the NHS and the increasing focus on the mentally disordered offender, later to be reflected through the deliberations and report of the Reed Committee.[1] The very act of creating us committed the powers-that-be to further change and action (even if occasionally their reactions were to be Frankensteinian as they recognised the extent and pace of change).

3.   We understood from the beginning that the SHSA was not an end in itself but part of a larger and longer process. Our work was to draw the special hospitals into the world of the NHS, to set goals and improve standards; other metamorphoses would follow which would use what we had done as a starting point. The hospitals had to be clinically and professionally acceptable before the process of altering service could sensibly be undertaken. It was, and is, essential to maintain a proper distinction between the three special hospitals (which are only today's vessels) and the high security service which is what they provide. That service still needs a clearer definition to assist its more appropriate provision, much of which in the future may be in different locations.

So we started in 1989, armed with experience, charged with enthusiasm and (blessedly) buoyed by ignorance. We pursued a set of definite initiatives to make change happen. These lay in management, clinical practice and professional values, the 'hearts and minds' of our staff, recognition of the patients, physical changes, standards and measurements, reaching out and openness.

---

1   The steering committee of the Review of Health and Social Services for Mental Disordered Offenders which was established in November 1990 and reported in November 1992.

MANAGEMENT AND LEADERSHIP

The SHSA, like most quangos responsible for managing organisations, had to be effective both by achieving and by protecting. Its demonstrable achievements gave strength to protect the hospitals from the predictable but unwelcome tentacles of the Whitehall octopus which sought involvement and control at inappropriate levels. The Authority-as-agency was both mirror and barrier since it had to reflect and shelter; but it had to get most things right to be allowed the luxury of protecting its hospitals and their vulnerability as they evolved. This paradox in power is not always successful, but it is workable.

> Mr Howard stays in his job. He remains Home Secretary for the same very good political reasons that put him there in the first place and kept him there at the last Cabinet reshuffle. Mr Lewis loses his job because a part of being Director-General of the Prison Service is to be a buffer for the political master. Since it is important for the future of the 'executive agency' system that the best possible candidates are attracted to its ranks, future candidates should note carefully what they are paid for. (*The Times* 1995)

We saw some of the inherent difficulties in this arrangement in 1995 with the prison service and the abrupt departure of its Director General over the question of where responsibility for managing the service lay.[2] When it does work, it enables leaders to lead publicly and managers to manage effectively.

If one accepts Rosemary Stewart's analysis of leadership in her book *Leading in the NHS* (1989), the special hospitals previously had not significantly or consistently moved beyond administration ('the carrying out of policies...being publicly accountable for doing so'). Leadership ('discovering the route ahead and encouraging and...inspiring others to follow') was not expected.

Under the umbrella of the SHSA, leadership and management could be established and thrive. From chief executive through (hospital) general manager to ward manager, a clear line of responsibility and authority was established and made personal. Although this adopted the reorganisation of management arrangements in the NHS proposed by Sir Roy Griffiths, it used it more explicitly and consistently. Individual objective setting and reporting at each level made the process of management sharply focused, extending into all aspects of each hospital. Many of the managers (particularly at the more senior levels) were recruited new to special hospitals and were intolerant of accepted practice. The sheer volume of new faces was in itself an important factor; mass made movement easier. The coherence of management effort, between executives and non-executives, HQ and hospitals, general manager and hospital team, was vital. Consistency in aims and challenges was essential to make headway against

---

2   See Derek Lewis' *Hidden Agendas* for a treatment of some of the difficulties.

an accumulation of cynicism, vested interest and ritualised practice. The existence of structures and strategies do not by themselves guarantee success. More recent events show that any relaxation of vigilance can lead to old problems recurring. The impact of ward managers – a hitherto unknown position in hospitals which had operated three different shifts with different charge nurses and (usually) different practices – was enormous, providing a key focus for staff and patients.

> ...one leader has given the wards the direction they needed. (SHSA 1993)

Before becoming intoxicated by the success of general management, it's important to note that, of course, not all managers were successful and that the harsh demands of difficult jobs produced high casualty rates. Many senior posts were filled two or three times during the Authority's brief life. Other managers who had faithfully served under the previous administration were unable to adopt new values and adapt to new techniques and had to leave, often unwillingly and with bitterness. General management sought to encourage and inspire but it also had the much needed capacity to make and enforce difficult decisions both in policy and over individuals.

REVIEWS AND RESULTS

In parallel with the management structure was a careful system of review of progress. On a personal level this meant that every manager was required to set objectives and report on progress to his or her supervisor. In organisational terms it required teams and their managers similarly to describe and quantify aspirations and report achievement, to the next level above. So the Chief Executive and SHSA itself annually met the Junior Health Minister with a formal agenda of targets and achievements and agreed the following year's tasks. The Chief Executive and HQ team met each general manager and hospital team twice yearly for discussion of written reports and the Chief Executive provided a critical summary of these sessions for the SHSA. A similar process went on within each hospital. This critical cascade recognised progress, probed weakness and confronted problems: within the organisation it made performance public and encouraged comparison both with previous performance and with other units. As a technique it was not novel but was particularly effective in the extent to which it was practised and in the thoroughness of its approach. It scoured every corner. By the way in which the outcomes were shared widely, it tested hard the objectives and scrutinised fiercely the judgements of success and failure. Importantly this was not an exercise *de haut en bas*, but goals mutually pursued; there were painful sessions but with a general recognition of lessons learnt.

STANDARDS AND MEASUREMENTS

Central to effective and sustained change were the careful definition of standards and the identification of relevant measurements which could be used to record progress. The cyclical pattern of standard setting, reporting, assessment and improvement is a basic management (and clinical) tool. Selecting the right standards and devising usable measurements is markedly more difficult. Frequently standards seem distant phantoms at ward level (paper generation to keep management happy) and some measurements were no more than proxies which did not immediately relate to the quality of care. We have all painfully learnt that it's easier to measure quantity than quality and subsequently had to assimilate the depressing message that numbers alone are one-dimensional and (often) misleading. The provision of psychiatric care and the assessment of progress or recovery in psychiatric illness do not neatly match obvious indicators used in the treatment of physical illness. Successful operations and healed wounds do not readily translate in terms of good mental health descriptors. Behaviour within the institution during stays measured in years, and its relationship to environment and available therapies are not easily matched: variables abound and observation and recording is usually limited, if not primitive. Extrapolating that process to observing behaviour outside the institutions and establishing causal links with hospital care seems even further away.

Nevertheless difficulty is no reason for not attempting. We deliberately, from the beginning, set standards, both general and specific; indeed the wide sweep and high ideals were usually precursors delineating the territory before more detailed expeditions which identified the salient features and related them to the whole. Broad policy statements were written on such key areas as nursing practice (1991), complaints (1992), control and restraint (1992), security and therapy (1992), environment (1992), seclusion (1993) and the Patients' Charter (1994). Each of these contained principles which were translated into specific standards.

A formal contract (or 'service level agreement') was prepared which grouped these standards and described the required reporting. In its final form, in April 1996, the contract covered these quality areas:

- Multidisciplinary teamwork and treatment planning
- The Patients' Charter
- Structured activity related to treatment plans
- Seclusion and management of disturbed behaviour
- Safeguarding safety (public, staff and patients)
- Implementation of 24-hour nursing care
- Clinical audit
- Standards of environment and patient accommodation

o Health of the Nation targets

o Implementation of Prison Service agreement.

Each area had four components: standard, indicator, target and return. A sample area would look like Table 5.1: (extract from 1995/6 senior level agreement, SHSA).

Table 5.1 Quality Standards 1995/1996

KEY QUALITY AREA Quality Standard	Indicator/ Measurement	Target	Return
1. Patients will have access to a minimum of 25 hours structured activity per week.	System in place for accurate recording and collection of information.		
	(a) Average hours provided per patient per week.	25 hours (minimum standard)	Average hours provision per patient per week.*
	(b) Percentage rehabilitation therapy/education/organised recreation sessions cancelled for non-therapeutic reasons.	not more than 5%	Percentage (and no.) sessions cancelled by category.*
	(c) Average hours actually available per patient per week (after cancellations)		Average hours actual availability per patient per week*
	(d) Average hours attended per patient per week		Average hours attendance per patient per week*
2. Structured activity will be designed to respond to needs identified through individualised treatment plans.	Demonstration of method of assessing patient needs.		Report
3. Structured activity linked to individual treatment plans.	Availability of appropriate activities responding to identified needs of ethnic minorities.		Report on plan and implementation.
	Availability of appropriate activities responding to the identified needs of women.		Report on plan and implementation.

The summarised report[3]on this area (for a six month period) was in this shape:

Structured Activity[4]

The provision of structured activity, linked to patient treatment plans, is central to the work of the special hospitals. It is of all the more concern, therefore, that performance in this area is well below the agreed quality standard at all three hospitals:

Table 5.2 Structured Activity

Agreed Standard = 25 hours/week

	Average hours provision / patient / week (a)	Sessions cancelled (b)	Average hours actual availability / patient/ week (c)	Average hours attendance / patient / week (d)
Ashworth	20.8	16 (5.1%)	19.5	10.2*
Broadmoor	13.59	186 (8.72%)	12.39	7.93
Rampton	17.92	5.3%	16.92	12.44

* 8.2 per cent of patients did not attend *any* activities. Of the 91.8 per cent who did attend, an average of 11.1 hours/patient/week is recorded.

The above table illustrates both the scale of under provision and the low level of take-up of activity provided. The best level of take-up is at Rampton Hospital; however, even then the attendance figures represent just under half the agreed minimum standard.

This level of performance is unacceptable. Measures will need to be taken at each hospital to:

o improve the level of provision available. It is important that the range of activities offered can be tailored to the clearly identified needs of individual patients and related to treatment plans.

o improve the level of take-up by patients

o identify reasons for non-attendance, including any common patterns or themes which emerge

o ensure that recording systems capture all structured activity, including that which is ward-based

3   This formed part of the Chief Executive's report to the SHSA in November 1995.
4   Refers to planned and organised sessions in the hospital specifically linked to the patients' care plan.

    ○ demonstrate significant progress towards achieving the minimum standard of 25 hours/patient/week in the next quarterly monitoring reports.

One of the major problems of balance was to seek enough information to be significant without attempting to be comprehensive and producing indigestible superfluity which, by its very bulk, is self-defeating. This is progress by beacons rather than by floodlighting, but the illumination must be sufficient to follow the chosen path.

The methodology was sound and tested and the ability to select appropriate measures was improving: the definitive criteria were, and are, some way off. This remains one of the most important areas for further work and requires explicit linking with carefully focused research projects to clarify and refine standards and to assess achievements.

PHYSICAL CONDITIONS

Slums do not encourage optimism or reward effort; while each hospital had, in 1989, some good buildings, that list was heavily outweighed by other areas sadly inappropriate for modern psychiatric care or for long-term asylum (both roles fulfilled by each Special Hospital). Significant capital investment was urgently required to change conditions, open opportunities and communicate to patients and staff vital messages about value and choice. Such investment needed to concentrate on patient areas and to be made on the basis of structured analysis of need which, in turn, meant defining our requirements. This important area is dealt with in more detail in Chapter Eight. While good conditions do not automatically ensure best practice their absence makes achievement less likely; to ignore the close relationship between working practice and working conditions is managerial hypocrisy. The improvement in morale and behaviour – of both patients and staff – after a refurbishment or new build was readily observable. Indeed the very act of moving a unit to new quarters could accelerate other changes.

CLINICAL PRACTICE AND PROFESSIONAL VALUES

Most staff in the hospitals were, and are, professionally qualified.[5] Many felt that the prevailing conditions in the late 1980s inhibited them, in professional terms, from using their skills fully and appropriately:

> Accepting that security is an essential and required element in Special Hospital life goes without saying. What remains a frustration however is the extent to which it constitutes an overwhelming and at times unjust and unexplained barrier placed deliberately in the path of progressive initiatives.
> (Brian Parry in the Ashworth Report 1992)

The first requirement was to acknowledge and welcome professions and their practitioners; the next to help them state, or restate, their standards and codes; then to provide a nurturing ambience; and finally to build the expectations thus generated into the daily reality of clinical life. This latter was summarised in each hospital's contract:

4.1 This section of the specification relates to those professions that contribute to direct patient care, including medicine, the professions allied to medicine, those deemed to be within the sphere of 'rehabilitation services', social work, and nursing.

4.2 It is key that there is an agreed common approach to service development and delivery, that meets organisational goals. It should be explicit and meaningful to all within the organisation. It will be based on a model of multi-disciplinary team-work and treatment planning, and will require an investment in continuing professional development; and the facilitation of excellence in clinical leadership.

4.3 Within the framework of multi-disciplinary work, and the drive towards systematic individual patient care, each profession will establish its own development agenda and standards, with a focus on clinical leadership that contributes to the management and business processes of the organisation. This will enable a contribution from the professions, through the clinical leader, to the vision, development, delivery and to the evaluation of services. This will facilitate the development of clinical teams and a move to determining outcomes.

---

5   In 1997, approximately 58 per cent of nursing staff are qualified and 42 per cent are nursing assistants. Ward staffing requires a radical review. The old notion of 'qualified' and 'unqualified' staff is anachronistic; there is no place in the special hospitals for unqualified staff. There is, however, a need for a rethink of the skills and qualifications required at ward level, based on the needs of individual patient groups. From such an analysis should emerge a new profile of ward staffing requirements which will be markedly different from current thinking; the introduction for example, of social therapists as employed in Holland may provide a response to both the needs of our patients and the general and increasingly difficulty of attracting nurses into psychiatry.

The approach to individual professions varied: for nurses, a statement of what was expected was required:

> To provide a skilled and committed nursing workforce, working in a partnership of care which recognises the needs of patients and respects their rights as equal members of society to choice, privacy and dignity.

> To uphold professional values and accept accountability for nursing practice within the multi-disciplinary team. (SHSA 1991)

This statement, elaborated and expanded within the strategy to cover all aspects of the nurses' work, was new to the hospitals. No such touchstone had previously been defined, nor had such expectations been set down. It provided the basis for assessing nurses as they practised and made clear to each nurse what was required of him or her. It also importantly made standards clear to the other professions within the hospitals.

Psychologists and social workers were encouraged to produce their own parallel statements. Particularly through the Royal College, psychiatrists were encouraged to describe and develop their role beyond the statutory 'Responsible Medical Officer'[6] minimum enshrined in the Mental Health Act.

In one particular situation a profession was newly introduced into the hospitals. In the major task of transforming the prison-type 'occupations' workshops into dynamic psychiatric rehabilitation units, occupational therapists were brought in and some existing staff sent off for training to become occupational therapists. These staff returned to their work with a marked difference in their approach and with much higher expectations in regard to care and therapy.

The cumulative effect of this was gradually to assert professional patient-focused values as the centre around which each hospital revolved. Paradoxically at the same time we were demanding of these professionals that they be territorially unselfish and combine in teams to take care for individual patients forward. This was, and is, a more taxing requirement: the switch from professional boundaries to professional confidence is a maturation process that does not come easily – the special hospitals are not alone in discovering this.

HEARTS AND MINDS

We faced a dual challenge: a number of the staff would oppose change and would want to maintain the status quo – which we saw as essentially untherapeutic – and with it their own position in power and habit. They were oppo-

---

6   In relation to a person liable to be detained in hospital, this means the registered medical practitioner in charge of the treatment of the patient.

nents. Many staff were potential allies but were cautious, even doubtful, about open support for change. They had seen other initiatives fail and other champions fall. They were sceptics. Their experience was illustrated at Ashworth Hospital in an extract from the 1992/3 inquiry which was set up to investigate the circulation of offensive literature:

> ...intimidation took four forms: personal confrontation, which was not common and rarely led to personal injury; damage to property but for which often the tangible evidence was not preserved; telephone calls for which there was never any evidence other than the victim's word; and mail, some of which had been retained but most had been destroyed. Some people had suffered spasmodically; some had suffered when feeling were running high at the time of industrial disputes; and some had been the victims of a sustained and prolonged campaign. The resilience and fortitude of the latter category was impressive.

Essentially our task was to disarm and redirect opponents (and if we could not succeed in that to remove them) and to convert the sceptics with consistent messages and practical achievements. In its most extreme and testing manifestation this process was demonstrated in withstanding the vicious industrial action in Ashworth and Rampton Hospitals just before Christmas 1990. More subtly the work was pursued through separate programmes in each hospital which sought to involve staff personally in setting the goals and to identify specifically and resolve areas of doubt or dispute. These approaches differed in style between the hospitals but shared three essential characteristics:

1. They were personally endorsed by the hospital's general manager and senior staff (for instance at Broadmoor Hospital this entailed the general manager and SHSA Chief Executive, among others, taking the 'hot seat' in open staff meetings to respond to any question or criticism concerning the changes).

2. A heavy focus on ward-based clinical teams (arranging 'away days' with facilitators to examine roles; sponsoring new approaches to multidisciplinary working and recording of achievements).

3. Hospital-wide communication which showed and explained change. Some of this was written material (newsletters and hospital magazines); some was through specific targeted groups led by change agents; some through representative bodies (made up of nominated individuals from wards and departments at Broadmoor Hospital); some by other devices such as an open (and anonymous) 'query line' where any question would be answered frankly.

The gradual shift to support could not be attributed to one initiative; rather it was cumulative. Techniques would be effective for a while and then need refocusing; so the Broadmoor comprehensive change programme had a life of about three years before standing down. The rate of conversion varied and other events revealed gaps and disappointments. Gradually, however, verified by monitoring and observations, behaviour and expectations changed, leaving negative attitudes still present but increasingly isolated. This remains a task unlikely ever to be completed: the nature of large institutions with their centripetal forces and the adverse pressures on those providing this service may at any time combine – if management is not vigilant and persistent – to allow a recrudescence of the negative. The volatile mixture of illness, crime and detention, always present in a special hospital, can quickly lead to serious incidents at any time. But, it needs to be remembered that one 'scandal' does not indicate the total failure of the system.

RECOGNITION OF PATIENTS

The same philosophy that encouraged staff to assert their professional values required that patients be seen as the centre of high security service rather than its raw material. The patient is a citizen detained. Detention does not obliterate rights but obviously imposes restraints; in detention, safeguards are even more important. The focus has to move from slogans ('the most dangerous men in the country', 'mad or bad') to a consideration of each individual. Once that shift was articulated it was axiomatic that the rights of patients needed to be considered and expressed – for example within the Patients' Charter (see Appendix 1) and the Complaints Procedure (where a novel and, to many staff, alarming feature was the acceptance that evidence from patients needed to be seriously considered). Equally, within the clinical sphere the active and personal involvement of the patient in the process of planning and monitoring treatment betokened a significant adjustment of the staff–patient relationship, away from the keeper and the kept, towards the genuinely therapeutic. This was not a naïve sprinkling of fairy dust, but a careful application of appropriate psychiatric practice. Some staff found this difficult, particularly if they had, consciously or not, despised patients because of the behaviour or offences that caused their admission. It is not only the patients who have to learn to live with what they have done; staff can feel a repulsion which will colour their practice if it's not understood and addressed.

The need to protect the patient within the institution was recognised from the beginning. The Mental Health Act Commission has understandably concentrated heavily on the Special Hospitals (see Chapter 18 for details of this) but within each hospital the SHSA set up a sub-committee (The Hospital Advisory Committee) with direct access to Chairman and Chief Executive. Interestingly the first chairmen of these bodies included a bishop, a QC and a blond-haired disc jockey! Primarily these bodies fulfilled the role of 'managers' under the Mental Health Act carrying out locally the process of review of detention. Their independence of local management added weight to their reviews. However, they also had a key role as 'eyes and ears', to visit freely, observe and report to the hospital general manager. This function did not normally involve dramatic findings but the committee's evidence was part of the new system of checks and balances, influencing and informing.

Even more specifically, a patients' Advocacy Service was created, initially at Ashworth Hospital and subsequently at Rampton Hospital. It was a totally separate service from the hospital although based within the campus, managed by another body (on Merseyside a Citizens Advice Bureau). It existed to support patients, pursue their interests and defend their rights. Deliberately, the creation of a group of patients' 'champions' emphasised a determination to view and treat patients with regard for their individual needs and rights. This was not achieved without some initial difficulties and, necessarily, some readjustment of attitudes. The verdict of the Advocacy Service at the end of their first year at Ashworth was:

> We would argue that in attempting to meet these objectives, since commencing full operations in January 1994, we have achieved very significant results. In working with patients we hope to have bolstered respect for their rights as individuals, whilst by reducing conflict we may also have helped the Hospital itself to run more smoothly and more effectively. (Ashworth Patient Advocacy Service 1994)

Another recognition of changing dynamics!

Closely linked in purpose was the establishment of patients' councils in each hospital. Although such bodies had existed elsewhere in the psychiatric service, they were new to the special hospitals where, given the literally enclosed environment and the long stays of most patients, their relevance was obvious. The purpose was straightforward: to create a representative group of patients who could air grievances, suggest change and speak directly to senior hospital staff on such matters. The evolution was more uncertain: election (or selection) offered its own problems given the instability of many patients and the manipulative tendencies of others. The councils benefited from tactful help from staff during their early days – nurturing the fledgling without dominating it (at Ashworth this role was later taken on by the Advocacy Service). The attendance by senior managers, hospital and headquarters, for question and answer sessions was an important ingredient in their development. As the Rampton Hospital Council (1994) said:

> Managers, clinical and other staff may at times have found it uncomfortable to hear what some patients have to say about the quality and sensitivity of the service patients receive. But, if we are really being encouraged to openly express our views and concerns in a safe atmosphere, and contribute towards achieving a change in the culture, then the least we should expect is

that those concerns be genuinely heard and where appropriate, prompt and effective action initiated. If not, any existing frustrations are further exacerbated, possibly leading to formal complaints and a further loss of management and clinical time. (pp.18–19)

Finally the patients' voice was expressed through their writing and publishing their own magazines which both expressed their own view of the hospitals and health professions (often in sharp satirical form) and offered an outlet for printing writing on other subjects.

Within the pages of the best established of these magazines, *The Chronicle* at Broadmoor Hospital, were printed the record of interviews between the editor and figures such as the chief executives of the SHSA and MHAC; John Bowis, Junior Health Minister; Jo Brand, comedienne; and David Brindle from *The Guardian.*

REACHING OUT AND OPENNESS

Complementary to changes inside the hospitals was the construction of effective and well-trafficked bridges to all manner of relevant organisations outside

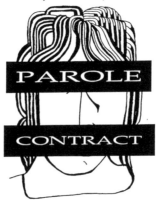

Figure 5.1 'Catch 22' from the Broadmoor patients' Chronicle

the walls. An important part of this was the encouragement to visit: from members of the royal family through politicians and health service leaders to journalists and practitioners in health and criminal justice and, simply, local residents. All were invited and welcomed, more especially if they had expressed negative views about the hospitals (usually, of course, uttered with the deepest conviction of sheer ignorance). Most visibly learnt; many were impressed; few remained scornful. MPs who inflated rapidly over local transgressions by patients could deflate gently in the face of the task and the staff's obvious dedication. Of course, the initial public declaration was rarely withdrawn but subsequent statements were often more tempered.

In formal terms, other authorities were invited to sign agreements with the SHSA about mutual responsibilities for patients. So each of the then Regional Health Authorities were approached to pledge themselves with the SHSA to a set of minimum standards with regard to patients: these covered assessment, admission and transfer procedures, waiting times and co-operation between clinical teams. Not all regions responded but with several (usually focused around the relevant medium secure unit) the agreement marked a recognition of the need for closer contact, and a requirement for a service to suit the patients' needs rather than the bureaucratic and geographical divisions of the NHS. Later, as the role of regions changed, agreements were made with relevant Trusts.

Parallel with this an agreement was negotiated with the Prison Service, concentrating on the same essentials, again to foster co-operation and to provide a better service. As one reviewer described this attempt:

> Although the agreement demonstrates that these two services are working
> for improvements, the specificities of such agreements paradoxically open
> up possibilities for much greater outside criticism and possible litigation.
> The agreement is therefore a bold move. (Meux 1995)

Results were uneven. In some prisons, governors and medical officers responded enthusiastically; the SHSA Chief Executive gave a presentation at the Annual Conference of the Prison Governors and strong links were forged with specific prisons (e.g. Holloway with Broadmoor Hospital). Other pressures within the prison service sometimes overshadowed our agreement.

With both services, health and prisons, behind the formal text seethed a whole stew of activity and contact, not all of it complimentary. Closer working meant closer scrutiny and more opportunity for criticism, particularly when practice fell short of aspiration. But this in itself was a helpful spotlight, ensuring that fewer dark corners remained unobserved. To be open to demonstrate and claim is also to be open to criticism and to acknowledge the need to improve.

One of the continuing difficulties was that once the formal process of approval for a move had been completed, practical difficulties in terms of finding the right location and appropriate supervision frequently delayed the move. Therefore, hospital staff were specifically designated to work with other agencies to facilitate transfers. This was effective but delays in movement remained a problem: a small (but decreasing) number of patients waited over a year for such a transfer, often being penalised by being seen as a lesser priority (since they were already in hospital care) than admission candidates from other sources (e.g. prisons and courts). This was unfair and unmerited and, in some cases, actually detrimental. Again the very process of liaison had a two-way effect informing both parties.

Links and exchange were fostered particularly with professional and representative bodies (Royal College of Psychiatry and Royal College of Nursing) and with the academic world (Chairs were established with Liverpool University and London University and close working in education and training with several other universities, particularly Sheffield Hallam, Reading and East Anglia). Research and study in the hospitals were fostered.

Change became evident.

REFERENCES

Ashworth Patient Advocacy Service (1994) *Ashworth Patient Advocacy Service Report.* p.2.

Ashworth Report, The (1992) *Report of the Committee of Inquiry into Complaints about Ashworth Hospital.* 1, p.145.

Meux, C. (1995) Editorial in *Criminal Behaviour and Mental Health.* 5, 1.

Mullen, P. (1996) *Criminal Behaviour and Mental Health.* 6, 1, p.40.

Pilgrim, D. (1990/1991) In Openmind No.48, December 1990/January 1991.

Rampton Hospital Council (1994) *Second Annual Report (Sept 93–June 94).* Retford: RHC.

SHSA (1991) *Nursing in Special Hospitals.* London: SHSA.

SHSA (1993) *Evaluation of Impact of Ward Managers in their First Year of Appointment.* London: SHSA.

Stewart, R. (1989) *Leading in the NHS.* London: Macmillan.

The Times (1995) 17 October.

CHAPTER 6

The Politics of Change
A Chairman Remembers
David Edmond

INTRODUCTION

'The next meeting will be held at Rampton Hospital and will be hosted by Lesley Teeman who is the Chairman of the Board'. With this innocuous announcement to the members of the East Midlands Region of the Confederation of British Industry (CBI) began my personal involvement with Rampton and later with the Special Hospital Service Authority, an organisation as yet undreamt of in mid-1985. At the time I was General Manager of John Player and Sons in Nottingham and had been involved in business for almost 16 years, always in the tobacco business but in a wide range of roles and in the USA, Ireland and the UK. At that time I was also contemplating taking early retirement and moving on to other challenges. Little did I realise how challenging they would be or that they would involve a difficult and unfashionable part of the nation's health services.

The CBI duly met at Rampton, a formidable campus of buildings on the flatlands of north Nottinghamshire, in sight of the vast power stations of the Trent Valley, and with its own boiler-house chimney, regularly used as a marker point for low-flying RAF jets to deafening effect. The meeting itself was not particularly inspiring but after lunch we undertook a tour of the hospital. For me that was a turning point as we passed through the intense security of the entrance and into the long main corridor with its double locked doors at 20-yard intervals and into the presence of so many dark-suited, peak-capped, and key-jangling 'warders', or so one thought as a newcomer. So claustrophobic was the atmosphere that one member of the party felt unable to continue.

It was when meeting the 'inmates', or patients as one soon learnt to call them, that I started to have an appreciation of the work being undertaken in this institution. In listening to the day-to-day challenges facing the staff who lived

24 hours a day, seven days a week, 365 days a year, and for many years, sometimes a whole lifetime, with these often dangerous, frequently difficult people, I realised what a tremendous amount of dedicated work was being undertaken there. I left profoundly moved and remember recounting in great detail the events of the day to my wife that evening.

CHAIRMAN OF THE BOARD

It was only several months later, when I received a telephone call from Lesley Teeman asking me if I would be interested in becoming the Chairman of the Board at Rampton, that I thought about it again. By this time I was close to my retirement date and was involved in Industrial Tribunals and intended doing some teaching work at Uppingham School as their Industrial Consultant. I was completely unaware of the history, structure and responsibilities of the board or the commitment required but I immediately agreed to go forward with the idea. What I heard in discussion with Lesley was the story of a hospital, isolated, paranoid, mainly as a result of media intrusion, managed at arm's length by the Department of Health in London and with the close involvement of the Home Office. The feeling one had was of an organisation that did a very necessary job with little outside recognition and an uncertain direction. Following an investigative television programme entitled 'The Secret Hospital' which thoroughly condemned the hospital's methods and management it had been decided to establish the Rampton Board in 1979. The board was to be chaired by an outside businessman with four non-executives with a range of medical, nursing, probation service, administration and social work skills. Also serving on the board were the Medical Director, Dr Diana Dickens, the Director of Nursing, Marion Hendry, and the Administrator Dereck Atha.

As I eventually discovered the Board was very much sandwiched between the Department of Health and the day-to-day managers of the hospital. Having spent 15 years on the board of the Nottingham Playhouse, including five as its Chairman, and having operated always in this sandwich mode I felt that I was up to the challenge of Rampton.

The ritual interview in London followed at the mausoleum-like Alexander Fleming House, in the Elephant and Castle, the then headquarters of the Department of Health, where I met Brian McGuinness, then the Under Secretary responsible for the Special Hospitals. Brian was a man dedicated to working for those with mental health problems (indeed he subsequently worked for Mencap after retiring from the civil service) but not really a business man in an organisational sense. He had the habit of always typing his own letters on an ancient typewriter with multitudinous white corrections. He chaired the Office Committee by which progress at the hospital was 'monitored', a process of unbelievable pedantry with, to my mind, a complete lack of determination to get things moving. As it only met at the hospital every six months the chasing of actions had to be seen to be believed as items slipped from meeting to meeting without apparent resolution or concern.

I was taken to meet the then Secretary of State for Health, Kenneth Clarke, whom I knew both as my local MP and also from his previous visits to Players. This obviously did not count against me and I was duly appointed and took up my post in mid 1986. I arrived at Rampton to be shown my office outside the secure area, with its appropriate thickness of carpet, its appropriate desk and, wonder of wonders, a bar.

In all my business life I had never had, nor would have in the future, an office bar but it had been decreed, I was led to believe, that the role of Chairman was equivalent to that of a Vice-Admiral and one was to be provided with the rights and privileges accordingly.

All wonderful stuff but an indicator of organisation stuck in a civil service past, very reminiscent of my days in the Overseas Civil Service in Africa with the same feel of permanence.

THE ATMOSPHERE AT THE HOSPITAL

On taking up the role at Rampton perhaps it was this feeling of lack of change that was the most striking difference from the world of business with which I was familiar. The hospital's affairs were managed expertly by the triumvirate of Dickens, Hendry and Atha but they were all of a parity reporting to 'bosses' in London with no one really in charge at the hospital though in general, even if not in fact, the Medical Director was seen as 'in charge'. This could and did lead to tensions which I tried to defuse from time to time. Similar arm's-length relationships existed for the psychologists and the social services departments. There was no real sense of future planning and the only major building project in hand at the time was the refurbishment of the boilers!. Absolutely typical when one understood that the control of the capital programme was in the hands of the late and unlamented PSA. We never ceased to be amazed at what could be quoted by the PSA for the simplest of jobs. Annette Nosquith, my non-executive with local government experience, was almost reduced to foaming at the mouth at the proposed charges for the simplest of items. Sadly we lacked the right to go for tenders to local builders.

The range of activities not the responsibility of the Board was quite unbelievable: no negotiation on salaries and terms and conditions of staff; no ability to change budgetary items; no control over staff numbers; and no ability to discipline staff. Although the bulk of staff were members of the nursing profession the majority belonged to the extremely militant Prison Officers' Association. The Royal College of Nursing was represented at a low level but was toothless in the face of the POA.

As the board had no negotiating role with the POA I undertook to have 'discussions' with their leadership to try to bring some sense of community to their activities but without great success. Their strength was built on a strong 'security is paramount' ethos and a complete resistance to any idea of change of practice.

Of particular concern to the board was the so-called 'long-day' shift system whereby staff worked alternate ten-hour days enabling many to hold down second jobs. It led to totally contrasting ward practices from one day to the next which was invariably most confusing to the patients. All attempts to change this system were met with ferocious resistance as the overtime generated sometimes doubled a staff member's salary.

What was fascinating in all this resistance to change was the level of professional dedication by the bulk of the staff. Rampton dealt almost entirely with patients in the categories 'mentally ill' and 'mentally handicapped' (later to be renamed 'learning difficulties'). There were few 'psychopathic disorder' patients except for those with a dual classification. This meant that many of the patients presented extremely difficult management problems with which the staff dealt with great fortitude in many of the more extreme examples. Staff turnover was low, almost too low by modern management theory standards, and sometimes up to three generations of a family would be on the staff at one time. With the presence of staff housing around the hospital this led to a very self-protective and tight community.

The consultants at the hospital were a law unto themselves, operating with no overall management control over work habits or practices and certainly no peer examination of effectiveness. There was a game played by one of the non-executive directors called 'hunt the consultant!' This was played on a Friday afternoon, usually with little success. Certain consultants were clearly not up to their role but Department of Health failure to act meant they remained in post.

The fabric of the hospital was plainly in need of much refurbishment with particular need to find ways of getting rid of the practice of 'slopping out'. This was the focus of the Mental Health Act Commission during their quarterly visits to the hospital but one about which the board could do little as it was then constituted.

One role given to the Board was that of 'managers' under the Mental Health Act which meant that they had to approve the continuance of detention of patients. Fortunately our medical non-executive Dr Julian Roberts was a great tower of strength in this role.

The examination of patient complaints was a responsibility taken very seriously by the board. The complaints system was managed by the Administrator but we monitored it. In order to assist ourselves in this task, and to improve Board visibility, I divided the ward areas between the members so that all members visited their areas each month and I, as Chairman, undertook to visit all other parts and to visit all wards over a period of time. This management by walking about did much to improve the visibility and effectiveness of the board.

As the hospital came within the responsibility of the Junior Minister within the DHSS we had flying visits from a number of incumbents over my three-year stay; Baroness Trumpington, Lord Skelmersdale, and Douglas Hogg, when junior in the Home Office, all visited and dined well in Rampton fashion but little seemed to result from such visits.

Each year an annual report was produced and presented in London usually with little comment except exhortations to 'continue the good work'. However the annual reports must have led the Department of Health to decide that, if a Board was a 'good thing' for Rampton then a Board would be a 'good thing' for the other hospitals. This really was a poor piece of thinking. The Rampton Board had been founded following the adverse publicity of the Secret Hospital Programme and was a result of the subsequent enquiry with the aim of making the hospital more open. Such situations had not arisen at the other three hospitals at that time. A mere contemplation of why Rampton had its Board would have led them to question this decision and avoid much of the angst that followed.

Two new Boards were established, one at Broadmoor, under a retired Vice-Admiral, and one for both Moss Side and Park Lane hospitals under a retired businessman. The setting up of this latter single institution for two hospitals which regarded themselves as totally separate, with no real contact (the keys to one did not fit the other), and which believed they had been promised continuing separation, despite contiguous sites, meant that from the start the Board in Liverpool had a torrid time. At Broadmoor the problems were more to do with the military style of the new chairman and his quite genuine questioning of the responsibilities of his board which he believed did not reflect those he had been recruited to undertake.

THE SHSA FOUNDATION AND CHAIRMAN'S ROLE

At about this time a change in personnel at the Department of Health meant that the Special Hospitals came under the wing of Cliff Graham, a man of extraordinary drive who had been working up to this time on the reorganisation of the National Health Service under Roy Griffiths. It soon became apparent that Cliff wanted to put into place a new method of running the three hospitals (assuming Liverpool to be one) and that this would involve the establishment of a body charged with their management totally separated from the Department of Health.

On one fascinating drive from Rampton to Newark to catch his train he outlined to me in his inimitable convoluted style his ideas and on reaching the car park asked, again in a convoluted way, if, were such an organisation to be formed, I would be interested in managing it.

I replied in the affirmative as it was just what I felt was needed to manage these large and (to my mind, though not to others) necessary institutions in an efficient and effective way for the benefit of all concerned. I heard nothing more until asked to a strange meeting at Stoke Mandeville Hospital with Cliff Graham, Jimmy Savile, the entertainer who at that time was deeply involved in helping to solve a building project problem at Broadmoor, James Collins, a retired Department of Health senior civil servant who subsequently served on the SHSA board, and other department officials. To this day I do not know why this strange meeting was held, though I suspect that Cliff Graham was using it to check out relationships. Not long after that I was officially invited to become the non-executive Chairman of this new body to be known as the Special Hospitals Service Authority.

The Authority was the first of the new-style bodies set up following the publication of the white paper 'Working with Patients' and was to be guided by six aims established from the outset. These were: to ensure the continuing safety of the public; to provide appropriate treatment for patients; to ensure a good quality of life for both patients and staff; to develop the hospitals as centres of excellence for training staff of all disciplines in forensic and other branches of psychiatry, psychiatric care and treatment; to develop closer links with local and regional NHS psychiatric services; and to promote research into fields related to forensic psychiatry. Looking at those aims today it is hard to realise what a tremendous change in emphasis they presaged.

At Rampton great efforts had been made to forge closer local links and over a considerable period of time they had led to the successful opening of one hostel for newly discharged patients in Nottingham shared with the charity Turning Point. But here were a set of statements challenging the hospitals to go much further, to become centres of excellence, to promote research, to ensure a quality of life. No wonder the new organisation started out with such enthusiasm.

Recruiting initially centred on filling the executive places on the Authority and I believe we were fortunate to obtain the services of Charles Kaye from Basingstoke as our Chief Executive. He brought the sort of vision and drive needed and with his extensive network we were able to recruit other outstanding people to the Board, Bob Hawkins as Finance Director, Frank Powell as Head of Nursing Services and Pamela Taylor as Head of Medical Services. I was ably assisted by four non-executives of wide experience in different fields, James Collier, whom I had met earlier, formerly Under Secretary of the Department of Health Mental Health division, Dorothy Barrett, a former director of the John Lewis partnership and former non-executive member of the Prisons Board, and two practising psychiatrists, Donald Dick, who in addition to his community work had served on the Broadmoor Board, and Jim Higgins, a practising forensic psychiatrist and former member of the Parole Board. We were all provided with a 250-paragraph guide on how to be an Authority!

EFFECTING CHANGES

The organisation believed it necessary to prove its independence by moving away from Alexander Fleming house, so premises were secured in Charles House in Kensington High Street. For political reasons the former staff from the Department of Health were offered the opportunity to refuse to move with us. One third did not want to move the short distance across the river, and those who did move were given two years grace within which they could ask to transfer back.

Sufficient numbers did move and operations started. When one looks back at the scale of the challenges and the achievements of the first four years of the SHSA's existence one feels a tremendous sense of pride. Think of the creation of a single hospital in Liverpool with its own name and shared identity, the creation of a 'corporate' business plan to map out the future direction of all three hospitals, the abolition of military-style uniforms for staff, the development of Ward Management to ensure 24-hour consistency of treatment of patients, the start of abolition of 'slopping out' by the provision of proper integrated toilet facilities and many more.

We were fortunate from a political point of view to be able to appoint General Managers to the three hospitals who all came from different backgrounds, medicine, nursing, and administration, thus demonstrating a lack of preference for any particular group within the professional politics of the hospitals. Our Ministers in the early years were immensely supportive; Roger Freeman and Stephen Dorrell both visited the hospitals to track progress. This is not to say that all was wonderful during this period, as the Ashworth Inquiry demonstrated. Sir Louis Blom-Cooper, an already avowed opponent of the Special Hospitals, conducted an inquiry into staff mistreatment of patients. That this led to the loss of the then General Manager was, in my view, a travesty of justice. It also demonstrated the continuing problems of a so-called 'hands-off' approach from the Department of Health which quickly reversed at the first sign of potential media problems.

The SHSA had to balance the needs of security with the need to liberalise regimes in three hospitals that had long remained in the shadows and been allowed to proceed in their own way. The developments undertaken to open up the hospitals meant that risks sometimes had to be taken against years of inbuilt attitudes within the hospitals. This did not always result in good relationships, particularly with the POA whose intransigence increased as each new development was proposed. So long as all remained out of the glare of publicity we were allowed to proceed, but when the media obtained leaked information about a particular development, as they so often did from domestic inaccurate or malicious 'deep throats' then issues escalated onto Ministerial desks very rapidly. Thus while initially political support for our activities was high I believe that latterly support began to wane as problems with the sort of patients we had in our care were not those desired by ambitious junior Ministers.

The increasing pace of change in the wider NHS started to spill over into the potential for developing the SHSA. Although we had been asked by Stephen Dorrell to produce a five-year business plan for the hospitals in 1992 which we duly did (after first carefully explaining to my Chief Executive what one was), the arrival of the internal market of purchasers and providers, the possibility of the establishment of independent trusts, care in the community, and the 'ring fencing' of the funding of the SHSA all led to changes in perception as to the future direction of the hospitals. This was also coupled with intense argument in the wider world of psychiatry as to the future means of seamlessly caring for patients nationally: how to place patients in the most appropriate therapeutic surroundings and be able to move them easily to less or more secure surroundings as required.

There were differences of opinion as to how to deal with seriously ill patients such as those in the hospitals where the average length of stay was eight years and where many patients stayed much much longer. The criminal justice system insisted on its right to send to special hospitals those it considered needed such care when it required to send them and was not moved to listen too carefully to arguments about appropriate catchment areas and the need to preserve beds for returning patients on trial leave.

The fact that the Special Hospitals did not charge originating authorities for the cost of the holding of 'their' patients made the movement of patients back to such authorities increasingly difficult in the face of tightening budgets. With great difficulty some of the first joint contracts were signed between regions and the SHSA to herald the start of new relationships.

Thus by the time I moved on from the SHSA in 1993 the world was changing. That my successors managed many of these changes successfully is apparent but we must never forget that the type of patient held in the Special Hospitals or their successors will always have the capacity to do the unexpected, to act unspeakably from time to time and one should always pay tribute to the men and women whose job it is to manage them on a daily basis 365 days a year. They are the unsung heroes and society should recognise the debt it owes them.

CHAPTER 7

Security and Therapy

Joy Kinsley

INTRODUCTION

The NHS Act, 1997, Section 4 states that the Secretary of State for Health is charged with the duty 'to provide and maintain establishments [in the Act referred to as special hospitals] for persons subject to detention under the Mental Health Act, 1959 (subsequently Mental Health Act 1983) who, in his view, require treatment under conditions of special security on account of their criminal propensities'. Although this duty is laid upon the Secretary of State for Health a considerable number of these patients who have been admitted through the criminal justice system may not be released without the consent of the Home Secretary. Thus two major government departments have interests in and responsibilities towards the running of the special hospitals. They may well have differing views on the security of those establishments and how it *affects* their specific interests. Indeed, they may even have different views on what the public interest might be. Unfairly perhaps, but none the less significantly, when James Saunders escaped from Broadmoor in 1991, it was the Home Secretary's resignation that the tabloid press howled for and not that of the Secretary of State for Health.

When the SHSA was formed in 1989, it was given two primary objectives:

1. To ensure the continuing safety of the public.

2. To ensure the provision of appropriate treatment for the patients.

Other objectives flowed from these, all important in their own right, but the maintenance of a proper balance between these two primary objectives inevitably provided the basis of the second major conflict, that between security and therapy. Which should come first? How many risks could justifiably be taken in furthering the patient's treatment? How was the public interest best to be served? The answers were often difficult; different viewpoints were argued passionately, and in trying to arrive at principles, the individual circumstances of patients could not be forgotten.

THE SITUATION IN 1989

Historically, the special hospitals had been managed by medical superintendents in much the same way as the old asylums. Those doctors had total responsibility for all that went on, but the specific task of security had always been largely the province of the nurses and very much an integral part of their training. They were, therefore, seen as gaolers as well as nurses. The greater emphasis on generic as well as forensic nursing training and on professional qualifications moved the situation on, but the majority of nurses still belonged to the Prison Officers' Association, who had represented them over the years, and this also tended to emphasise the custodial element of their role.

However, in security terms the link with the Prison Service was a natural one, especially as there was a relative lack of knowledge of the required level of security in the health service. Indeed, what inspections of security had been carried out in recent years had been done by the Prison Service, who for their part generally lacked the expertise in forensic psychiatric treatment and the situations it brought about in the Special Hospitals. The nurse in charge of security at each of the hospitals attended the annual conference of prison security officers and derived some support from this network. The advent of the SHSA in 1989 brought a different style of management with different expectations and an emphasis on new professional and more health service oriented ideas. These particularly affected the nurses who were carrying the main burden of security. Yet there had never been any specific training in security methods and awareness after the initial introductory training and too often professionally qualified staff, who may well have been entirely new to the situation, were expected just to know about these things. One might almost say that these were 'learnt at Nellie's knee'. In these circumstances it is not surprising that old ideas had been adhered to slavishly when no training programmes had been offered on the impact of developing therapy regimes on the basic principles and practice of security methods.

THE SHSA

As the SHSA director responsible for advising on security matters, I was asked to write a fundamental philosophy of security setting out principles on which future policy could be set. It was felt strongly that security was the responsibility of all staff and each individual member of staff must have a commitment to it. This security document entitled 'Security in the Special Hospitals – A Special Task' was drafted in a way which set out the principles clearly, simply and unequivocally. Although necessarily broadbrush, it came to be used as an important policy statement and was one of the building blocks for subsequent and related policies. The general managers were asked to ensure the issue of this policy statement to all members of staff so that there could be no doubting the Authority's stance in these matters.

A PHILOSOPHY OF SECURITY

The maintenance of a proper balance between the twin concepts of security and therapy is a very special task and a vital one. It is at the heart of the existence of the Special Hospitals. If either concept outweighs the other, it usually indicates that somewhere, somehow, the operation is out of kilter and becoming dysfunctional. In these circumstances the organisation will not work effectively.

On first examination security and therapy appear to be diametrically opposed, but in attempting to treat patients who are a 'grave and imminent' danger to the public, both are necessary and for treatment to succeed there must be, at the very least, a sense of security and safety. Realistically, the treatment of these patients cannot succeed without a strong and well-defined system of security which protects not only the public at large, but also staff, patients and all those who have to visit the hospital in whatever capacity. Security is, of course, fundamentally linked to 'dangerousness'. Part of the problem is that this is a variable state even for a single patient and there will be many changes in the state of dangerousness as treatment progresses.

In the *Health Service Journal* of August 1991, Charles Kaye, the SHSA Chief Executive said: 'Dangerousness is reduced as progress is made towards stabilisation and recovery, and treatment is thus part of security'.

To complicate matters further the public perception, and indeed that of other agencies, may be slow to accept that any change has taken place. The significant factor to them is always the nature of the incident and the likelihood of repercussions. In the situation where mental disorder has led to a serious offence or offences taking place, there are many who find it very difficult to allow that retribution is not always an appropriate part of the resolution or the best way of dealing with guilt. Obviously in dealing with a large number of patients in one hospital, however specialised it may be, security becomes a complex and dynamic state. Assessing risk has become much more systematic and hopefully accurate, but the real problem comes in managing the risk. Even allowing that treatment is a continuing process, which must be able to convey hope, progress can be very slow for some patients and the level of their dangerousness to society is such that long periods and release must inevitably be a long way off.

Early in its life the SHSA adopted the position that security and therapy were not separate entities. The guiding principle was that the most effective form of security lay in the treatment of the patient. All patients in the Special Hospitals are by definition treatable. It is, therefore, a primary aim to reduce the dangerousness of the patient by the use of all the methods available in modern forensic psychiatric practice and to provide containment in appropriate circumstances to the point when the patient may be safely released to the community or, more usually, to a less secure therapeutic environment.

Security will be achieved by a variety of means. It needs to be multidisciplinary and the responsibility of all staff. The various specialisms and clinical disciplines will obviously have different contributions to make, but none must avoid their own individual responsibilities and accountability. This involves being able to identify unacceptable risks and to understand and accept the remedial action which needs to be taken. The core value for security is contained within the professional relationships between staff and patients and the differing elements of the treatment programmes. This is a dynamic process, which can best be described as relational security.

RELATIONAL SECURITY

This begins with the patient and is essentially concerned with detailed knowledge of the patients and their situation and develops through the sound professional relationships that are essential in good psychiatric care. It will extend to relationships and professional agencies outside the hospital, so that although the institutional boundaries are very definite, effective security can start in the patient's own community situation. The centre of this network of close knowledge must be the consultant psychiatrist responsible for the patient together with that patient's primary nurse. The clinical team provides the ward context and radiates outwards through other departments and managers. In specific security terms it relates to the security department and, either directly or indirectly, to the general manager.

Security matters may not always be at the top of senior management's agenda when all is going well, although it is such an essential element that it cannot be allowed to drop too far down the list of priorities. It is all too easy to be lulled into a false sense of security when all is quiet, but when things go wrong as they sometimes do and there is a serious breach of security, then apart from any other considerations, public reaction will bring it very firmly to the top. It is, therefore, a critical issue and one that must be safely dealt with for the hospital to retain credibility.

PHYSICAL SECURITY

Each of the Special Hospitals has to conduct their business within an envelope of secure conditions. This means that there must be effective physical barriers to prevent escape should there be an attempt to do so. This will include walls and fences, possibly both, to agreed standards. There will also be good lighting systems and other electronic aids such as closed circuit television cameras. The science and technology of the modern security industry is, of course, available to hospitals and just how much of this to use will be a matter of policy and decision. The Special Hospitals are commonly referred to in the media as prisons. This is usually in times of crisis, or that which is perceived as a crisis by the media, and certainly adds to the drama. However, they are not prisons but secure hospitals and there are a number of important differences. The objects of these institutions are not the same and the risks and pressures they have to deal with are different.

Prisons exist primarily to carry out the sentence of the courts. Their first objective must be the safe custody of the prisoners. Treatment or training are desirable objectives but not an essential part of the regime as in the Special Hospitals where it is the whole reason for their existence. Generally speaking, the prison population is predominantly male, young, active and not suffering from a recognisable mental disorder which can be modified by medical treatment. Prisoners are more likely to combine together to cause disruption and are subject to an internal system of discipline, which allows governors to punish those who break the rules.

There is no such disciplinary structure in the Special Hospitals. This can make it considerably more difficult to control those patients suffering from personality disorders which may or may not be complicated by mental illness. This is particularly so when they are grouped together in significant numbers in accommodation. The regime in Grendon Underwood Prison, which is dedicated to group psychotherapy and is the most comparable situation to the personality disorder units in the Special Hospitals is, therefore, much more structured. Although at Grendon treatment is a primary objective and the prisoners have all consented to take part in that process, the combination with prison rules and conditions allows for swift reaction to abuse of the regime by inmates (patients). Consequently although their security needs have much in common, it would be wrong for the Special Hospitals to simply imitate prison systems. In the hospitals the provision of good basic security and associated systems should provide the possibility of a relatively relaxed regime within those boundaries. A properly structured environment, reasonable living conditions and a system that is both fair and humane will go a long way to ensuring that security risks are reduced rather than exacerbated, but it has to be a system that is essentially within the Health Service.

Physical security should give an impression of strength and safety rather than overwhelming security. Sensitive landscaping can be used to reduce the impact of strong barriers. The overall design should, as far as possible, give the impression of a community or village life thus enhancing some of the social aspects of therapy and aiming to reduce some of the more harmful effects and isolation of detention. The provision of education, rehabilitation and pastoral facilities as well as leisure and social activities all have an important part to play in the provision of a safe environment. It is in this context that arrangements can be made for patients to be allowed appropriate forms of freedom which, if successful, may be gradually increased. Ultimately, such matters as leave of absence will have to be considered. Initially, the patient will be escorted or accompanied either in the hospital or outside it. If this is successful, there comes the question of allowing the patient to be unescorted at certain times and so treatment should progress. In the case of restricted patients (i.e. those for whom the Home Secretary's consent is necessary for release to be contemplated), it will be necessary to obtain Home Office clearance for these activities. The whole process must of necessity involve some risk, but it may be an essential part of progress and should in the end offer a better chance of a safe release to the community. The risk factor needs to be assessed on an individual patient basis and all patients, restricted or otherwise, need to have the same care and consideration applied to the process of risk assessment and management. In the final analysis the overriding factor must always be the maintenance of public safety.

PROCEDURAL SECURITY

In addition to physical security and relational security, there is a third system, which is perhaps the most tedious for staff to implement and that is best described as procedural. This is the methodology or means by which patients are managed and safe security maintained. These systems must be known, understood and accepted, as unobtrusive as possible and totally reliable. They should be derived from policy statements and expressed through clearly written operational instructions. They will include the various necessary regular checks on physical security: a system of security information reports and collation; reception and screening of goods and people going into the hospital; searching of patients; and checks in other areas right through to the provision and deployment of safe staffing levels and techniques for the control of aggressive behaviour. However, it always needs to be remembered that any system is only as good as the people who operate it. The Special Hospitals are very much in the 'people business' and systems, important as they are, can never be fully efficient without the application of sound judgement by the staff concerned. Similarly, it will be necessary for managers to be regularly reviewing procedures and adapting them when necessary to fit the changing circumstances of a dynamic situation.

DESIGNING FOR SECURITY

At the same time that this work was being developed I was able to work with John Lynch, an architect closely associated with prison design who had assisted the Woolf Inquiry into the severe disturbances at Strangeways Prison in 1990. His design for buildings and systems was definitive and of great importance to the Special Hospitals and other secure hospital units. John Lynch has the advantage of being a professional artist as well as an architect and he has a quite exceptional way of graphically presenting difficult concepts in an understandable and acceptable manner.

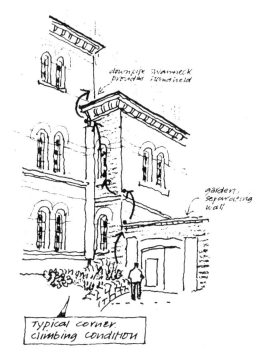

Figure 7.1 Security drawing by John Lynch

His work was crucial in trying to resolve yet another major area of conflict for the Special Hospitals, that is that the buildings tend to resemble a prison rather than a hospital. The physical environment is obviously very important and necessarily has to present a secure envelope, but there are ways in which the visual impact of security can be modified and offer a less stark and more acceptable image for a hospital. The use of the right materials, planning which encourages a sense of community and thus helps to reduce aggression and imaginative landscaping are all vital ingredients.

ESCAPES, ABSCONSIONS AND DISTURBANCES

The prospect of mental illness or disorder combined with dangerousness provokes fear in the public mind and ambivalence about the treatment of the individual patients concerned. None of this is helped by sections of the press which often choose to emphasise the sensational aspects of incidents. Patients are referred to as inmates and their nurses as guards. Television programmes will, for instance, often show pictures of old buildings instead of the new, although recent pictures are readily available to them. This is not to minimise the importance of escapes and it has to be recognised that the escape of John Straffen from Broadmoor in 1952 and the subsequent murder of a child by him does still strike fear into the local community if things go wrong. Rather it is to illustrate the highly charged atmosphere that can exist and to recognise and acknowledge the critical importance of the work of the Special Hospitals and the decisions that staff are called upon to make, often routinely. Conversely, the Blom-Cooper Inquiry into matters at Ashworth Hospital showed unacceptable standards in the treatment of detained patients and this provoked public anger and disquiet. All this serves again to illustrate the ever-present conflict between illness and dangerousness, therapy and security.

Escapes were defined as occurring from within one of the hospitals and they were differentiated from absconsions, which were described as occurring whilst the patient was outside the secure environment of the hospital or failed to return from some sort of temporary release. Some escapes occurred, notably at Rampton and Broadmoor, and all three hospitals suffered from situations of relative insecurity, disorder and home leave failures. James Saunders escaped from Broadmoor twice: once by using a file obtained from a workshop to file through window bars and once by scaling the perimeter wall by climbing a television mast which had been installed too close to the wall. Paul Marshall escaped from Rampton also through a window at night following failures of supervision. Disciplinary action against staff ensued, but the failures are often not only the fault of individuals but of the team as well. Invariably some other corrective action was shown to be necessary to protect and enhance the security systems. Nevertheless, it can be truly said that 'you are as secure as your weakest link'. A disquieting thought, but one that emphasises again how critical the professionalism and care of every member of staff is in these situations.

In 1992 there appeared to have been an excessive number of absconsions from outside escorts and these were the subject of a detailed examination. There were a number of common factors and these were addressed. There were a small number in which the degree of risk in relation to the activity proposed appeared not to have been adequately assessed and these gave added impetus to the work on risk assessment already being undertaken and its practical implications. But, typically, the absconsions were opportunistic actions which occurred following a lowering of supervision when, for example, a patient asked to use a toilet. In these sort of instances the patients were quick to take advantage of any lack of awareness by staff. Rehabilitation trips outside the hospitals, whether by individual patients or by small groups of patients escorted by staff, are important if the patient's reaction to the outside community is to be assessed with any degree of accuracy. These may include visits to shops or a locality of interest. The trouble comes when insufficient thought is given to the appropriateness of the location or to the possible effect on the public. Refreshments may have to be taken but it became necessary to curtail stops at public houses or visits to crowded town centres. On the other hand it is useful, some would say necessary, to know the reaction of a patient who has previously abused alcohol to being in that sort of environment following a period of treatment. Similarly, a patient who is being prepared for release after years of detention needs to be able to get used to crowded places again. There are no easy answers, but the policy was that all rehabilitation trips should have a carefully thought-out objective, risk analysis and a practical plan with clear instructions for staff to follow.

From all this came a recognition that risk assessment needed to become a more formal process and to be approached in a more rigorous and systematic manner. As the process developed it became clear that merely assessing risk was not enough and that the more important aspect was the management of the risk once the nature of it had become established.

SECURITY – AN INTEGRATED SYSTEM

An integrated system of security has been described in which all the professional disciplines have a stake. This still leaves the nurses as responsible for the greater number of the practicalities of the system. In some countries security staff are a separate group from the therapy staff. The duties in the reception area, patrols, searches or perhaps any necessary application of physical force to restrain a violent patient may be carried out by a separate specifically trained security staff. The case for this was carefully considered, but it was felt that really effective security must stem from detailed professional knowledge of the patient and that to take the other view does not allow sufficient weight to be given to the reality of security and the necessity for detention as an inherent part of forensic psychiatric practice. It is, in effect, an important tool to be used as part of treatment and according to need.

FINALLY...

It has been said that the Special Hospitals are different to prisons and this must clearly be seen to be so. The hospitals exist to treat patients and not merely to contain them. The philosophy and culture must be that of the National Health Service. They are different from other psychiatric hospitals and even regional secure units by reason of their heightened security measures. There are strong and inevitable links with the Home Office, but nevertheless the Special Hospitals are and must be seen as places for the treatment of sick patients. To achieve the apparently conflicting aims of therapy and detention calls for the very highest order of forensic psychiatric skills and deserves management of a similar order. The difficulties are clear, but the satisfaction of helping the patient and protecting the public can also be high and deserves recognition.

CHAPTER 8

The Physical Environment

Roger Hinton

THE PHYSICAL ENVIRONMENT'S CONTRIBUTION TO CARE

By convention and tradition, the design of prisons, workhouses, barracks, psychiatric hospitals and other large institutions has generally reflected a 'control' culture. Fences, locks, dormitories, large and impersonal halls, long corridors, high ceilings, acres of cream emulsion, institutional furnishings and an absence of any personalisation of private living space. These have become the firmly established hallmarks of a culture concerned with the 'management' of large numbers of people. Such depersonalising aspects of institution design are incompatible with the nurturing functions of growth and self-healing but in past years most of them were to be found within the special hospitals.

BREAKING THE MOULD

One of the SHSA's tasks was to normalise, as far as possible, the hospital environment in which people live and work; to minimise the impact of traditional 'hard architecture' and generally to ensure that the message conveyed and reflected by the built environment is one of care rather than custody, but without jeopardising security.

It is neither possible nor desirable to design secure psychiatric hospitals entirely without restrictive elements, but it is possible to ensure that design complements rather than frustrates the treatment process. The act of custody and the design of the buildings from which it is provided should not generate their own pathology.

THE BUILDINGS

The majority of the SHSA's building stock was constructed in the heyday of the large institutions. **Ashworth Hospital** is a composite of three sites constructed in different periods, whose buildings exhibit quite diverse characteristics. Ashworth South, formerly the Moss Side hospital, was opened in 1910 as the first 'State Institution for Mental Deficiency' – for people whom we would describe today as having learning difficulties. Here the emphasis was on secure building envelopes – with bars on the windows and locks on the doors – and with a low level of perimeter security. By contrast, Ashworth North, formerly Park Lane hospital, is the late twentieth century's major addition to high security hospital building stock. Completed in 1980, its construction followed a decision some ten years or so earlier to provide increased capacity in order to relieve overcrowding at Broadmoor Hospital. It was designed as a purpose-built high security hospital and is girdled entirely by a 5.2 metre concrete wall complete with anti-climb head. It comprises dispersed villa-type ward accommodation with centralised recreation, rehabilitation, education and sports facilities. The Ashworth east site comprised a collection of single-storey wards, completed in the mid 1930s. These were of a simple, perhaps primitive design, but each, having been built round a central courtyard, offered considerable scope for redevelopment.

Broadmoor Hospital was designed by Sir Joshua Jebb, architect of Pentonville Prison. It was completed in 1863 and at the end of the following year housed 309 patients. Large, three-storey Victorian ward blocks contrast sharply with a low rise two-storey complex commissioned in 1990 to provide 115 beds, new entrance building, administration block, central stores and catering facilities. Facilities for rehabilitation, recreation, communal activities and visiting are centralised.

The 300-bed core of **Rampton Hospital** in rural North Nottinghamshire was opened in October 1912 as Rampton Criminal Lunatic Asylum with the transfer there of 128 patients from Broadmoor Hospital. A further 85 patients were transferred in the following year. Its capacity was increased in 1921 with the opening of the first villa. The design was deemed so successful that, with modification, others followed in the period 1928–32, bringing the hospital's capacity to 1200 beds on a 190-acre site. Its design features five massive, three-storey ward blocks linked to offices, recreational facilities and workshops. There are two separate villa areas and a further discrete re-socialisation area comprising four villas. This dispersal of villas into smaller, natural groupings is a most successful aspect of the site's design.

THE SCALE OF THE CHALLENGE

At the time when the SHSA was set up, the hospitals operated in something of a vacuum in estate planning terms. Little was known about the condition of the estate. There were no up-to-date Development Control Plans for the three sites, nor was there an objective basis for establishing investment priorities. Existing

Building Notes and Design Guides were not relevant to the unique requirements of the special hospitals.

The challenge for the SHSA was to take stock of the estate which it had inherited, develop a set of contemporary building standards and apply them to a heterogeneous collection of buildings in a way which would assist in implementing the Authority's priorities.

A period of ordered introspection was needed as a prelude to the construction of investment programmes aimed at effecting a determined cultural shift away from the institution and towards individual recognition and care. During the three years which followed, that programme involved:

1. The preparation of a set of Environmental Standards – minimum, patient-centred standards with which all wards would comply.

2. An audit of each of the 79 wards across the three Special Hospitals against these new standards.

3. Translation of deficiencies identified into an investment programme.

4. The completion of Development Control Plans for each of the hospitals.

5. The development of a Ward Design Guide to inform all future upgrading and redevelopment work, addressing aspects of therapy and security in a way which recognised their complementary nature.

6. The introduction of commercial procedures for the control and reporting of cost, timing and quality of the overall capital programme and its component schemes, and competitive commercial practice for design and construction.

In reviewing extant plans for building development, the SHSA decided, with one exception, not to pursue those involving massive building 'complexes', in favour of a co-ordinated programme of smaller, discrete schemes whose content and interrelationship were determined by an estate control plan for each site. Benefits included:

- o Greater flexibility, particularly in response to changes in therapeutic approaches and availability of funding.

- o Manageability – the projects are less vulnerable to cost escalation and programme slippage; individual components are more manageable.

- o The more rapid design and construction of individual components increases the prospect of those staff and patients involved in design actually still being around to occupy the building. The result is a greater commitment to the building and the real prospect of its being operated as intended.

o The phased approach enables designers of later phases to benefit from the experience of those designing and operating earlier phases; the benefits of hard-won experience can be incorporated.

The one exception referred to above related to the construction of the new three ward, 75-bed 'B' Block at Rampton hospital. When the SHSA came into being, plans for the replacement of 'B' Block by a large structure of similar, conventional design, employing heavy construction methods, were well advanced. The new authority took an early decision to continue with these plans through construction, and the new 'B' Block was completed at a cost exceeding eight million pounds and occupied in 1992.

This decision was taken, however, only after a lengthy examination of the options of refurbishing the ward block as opposed to constructing anew. 'A' Block, of similar age, scale and design to 'B' block, had recently been the subject of a major and lengthy refurbishment programme. In the event, the scale and complexity of the work had been underestimated and whilst the result was successful, it was likely that an invitation to tender for a similar upgrading of 'B' block would, in the light of the recent 'A' block experience, result in a substantially higher tender price. This, taken together with the comparative cost of a new building and the risks of the unforeseen inherent in the refurbishment of any old building, particular one of this scale, weighted the decision in favour of new build.

The 'B' Block wards continue to operate successfully and provide a pleasant modern living environment. But in hindsight, one cannot help but wonder whether an opportunity was missed to depart from the ward block aspect of institutional culture and to employ the money, energy and creativity of the designers on something more imaginative. Our later investments were channelled in that direction.

During the seven years of the SHSA's existence five new wards were constructed – three on the Rampton Hospital site to replace those in the time-expired 'B' block, and two new wards constructed on the Ashworth Hospital east site – to replace those lost with the closure of the hospital's south site. The majority of the ward transformation was, however, achieved through the conversion and upgrading of existing building stock.

THE CORNERSTONE – ENVIRONMENTAL STANDARDS

Recognition of the importance of developing ward environmental standards emerged from the confluence of several themes. Firstly, there was a need to evaluate the newly constructed, 115-bed first phase of the hospital's redevelopment. Added to this was the government's value for money drive. A culture was rapidly taking root in the NHS which recognised that the scope for upgrading existing buildings had not been fully exploited. A rational basis for constructing a refurbishment programme was essential.

1992 saw the development by the SHSA of a set of ward environmental standards – minimum standards with which all current and future wards should comply. The standards themselves were not technical standards. They were user-oriented, reflecting a belief in the primacy of personalised delivery of care and a rejection of the institutional. Draft standards were prepared in collaboration with hospital staff and patients. The need to replace dormitories with single rooms complete with en-suite toilets and washing facilities came top of the agenda.

The standards themselves were classified as either primary or secondary, and are set out in Table 8.1 below. Primary standards were assigned a higher weighting to reflect their importance.

Table 8.1 The SHSA's Ward Environmental Standards: 1992

Primary Standards

Standards which any new build or upgrade should incorporate:

1. Single room accommodation
2. Elimination of 'slopping out'[1] either by provision of en-suite facilities or night-time access to toilets.
3. A patient call system installed in each room
4. A maximum size of 20 beds in general wards and 12 beds in special care wards
5. Private interview space where patients can meet visitors, solicitors and other advocates.

Secondary Standards

Standards which are highly desirable:

1. Private dressing/undressing facilities
2. Access to fresh air and daylight
3. Ready patient access to storage facilities for personal effects
4. Provision of staff call system to enable staff to summon assistance
5. Adequate space for on-ward therapeutic and recreational activities
6. Designated smoking and non-smoking areas
7. Personal room lighting switches which are readily accessible to patients
8. Attractive décor and furnishings
9. Good quality dining facilities.

These minimum standards challenged conventional institutional practice and ushered in suitably 'modern' design principles: the elimination of dormitories,

---

1 The process whereby patients use a chamber pot for night-time toileting, and queue to empty it at the ward toilet the following morning.

over-sized wards and 'slopping out'. Patient-operated nurse call systems were to be introduced to all wards. Individual bedroom lighting controls, proper accessible space for the storage of personal property, private interview space and designated smoking/non smoking areas featured in all subsequent new-build and upgrading schemes. Attention was to be paid to improving standards of decoration and furnishings and dining facilities. Professional interior design consultants were drafted onto project teams to bid goodbye to an era of cream-and-green emulsion, linoleum floored corridors and orange plastic-covered armchairs.

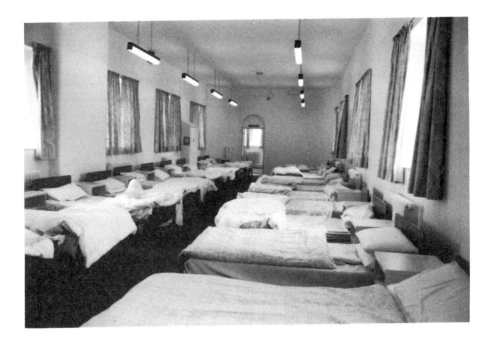

Figure 8.1 Dormitory, Weymouth Ward, Broadmoor Hospital

Each ward in the three Special Hospitals was audited for compliance with these new standards. A management summary for each hospital was distilled from these detailed findings, describing the main problem areas identified across each site and the position with regard to each ward. Finally, it ranked the wards according to their scores and classified them as either low, intermediate or high quality wards.

Future ward investment priorities were informed in large part by the results of that audit and 1993 saw the introduction of the first investment programme aimed at eliminating the worst features of special hospitals' wards. By March 1996, just three years after commencement of the ward upgrading programme:

- the number of high quality wards had been increased in the same period from the original 33 to 64 (out of a total of 76 wards)
- all of the 24 wards formerly classified by the audit as being of poor quality had been upgraded and subsequently reclassified as being of either medium or high quality.
- the number of dormitory beds had been reduced from 316 to just 62.

But the scale of the change tells only part of the story. The newly upgraded wards were deemed by patients, staff and outside observers to be functional and attractive. Wards reported on the favourable response from patients and staff to their new surroundings. Importantly, the transformation of these wards paved the way for the introduction of 24-hour nursing care. This could not have taken place without the programmes of work to reduce overcrowding and introduce call systems, privacy locks, facilities to permit a wider range of therapeutic and recreational activities to take place on the wards and modern sanitary facilities.

The process of reducing ward overcrowding and the installation of integral sanitation in patients' rooms did, however, generate a need for additional revenue and it was this as much as anything else which constrained the pace of change. Reducing the number of patients housed in each of several wards creates a demand for more staffing. Thus reducing the size of each of four 25-bed wards to 20 beds generates a need for an additional fifth ward, complete with a team of staff to run it.

Following adoption of the new environmental standards in 1992, all ward upgrading and conversions made provision for integral sanitation. Its introduction by the 'three into two' approach whereby a single patient room is converted into two en suite toilets, each of which serves an adjacent room, reduced ward bed capacity by one third with a corresponding increase in the number of beds to be found elsewhere to maintain the same level of patient capacity – a significant practical difficulty. The adoption of 24-hour care in 1995 obviated the need for en suite sanitation and rendered that standard obsolete.

DESIGN GUIDE

A determination to modernise and de-institutionalise the hospitals' wards and, where desirable, to replace them, begs a number of questions which precede the design process.

What functions do we want the wards to serve? How do we want them to be organised within the ward? Should we adopt design and material standards appropriate to a 'generic' ward which can cater for any type of patient but is expensive and over-restrictive for some? Should we strive for a design which is specific to the needs of a nominated group of patients – it may be more economical to provide but lack longer-term flexibility. What are the respective pros and cons of single and two-storey wards? Why have special hospital wards traditionally been so expensive to construct in relation to other types of ward? Are some of the design and materials standards employed inherent in the design of a secure ward or simply unchallenged perpetuation of past practice?

The SHSA commissioned the services of John Lynch, a design consultant with extensive experience of both secure design and its relationship with therapy, to work with special hospital staff in the preparation of a Secure Ward Design Guide (SHSA 1992) specific to the needs of the high security hospitals and which addressed these and other issues. The Ward Design Guide was published in April 1992 and formed the basis of all subsequent conversion and new-build work. Its starting point was a detailed examination of the role played by the ward in providing both a home for patients and a focus for treatment. It examined the philosophy of and interrelationship between the ward and other hospital departments together with aspects of security, in terms of both the design of the ward itself and its relationship with overall site security. It provided advice on design concepts, model schedules of accommodation, room data sheets and standards of space, materials and engineering, together with cost standards. The aim was not to prescribe a 'standard' ward, but rather to provide basic information applicable to a number of situations, to inform the work of project and design teams and set minimum standards.

INTERIOR DESIGN

Good interior design is a key to creating an attractive, relaxing, non-institutional setting in which treatment can take place and is of vital importance for Special Hospital patients, for whom the ward will be their home for many years. This aspect of design had been sadly neglected in the past. One specific aim was to involve both patients and staff in the process, to give the former the opportunity to personalise their own private living space and involve them in creating the overall ambience of the ward. The design of all wards, both upgraded and new, should feature the work of specialist interior designers with relevant experience.

The marked benefits of this approach far outweighed the modest costs involved. The careful use of colour, texture and fabrics can transform a bleak, institutional setting into a home. An impersonal, barren room can be transformed into a personalised bedroom. It is also apparent that where patients are involved in the interior design process and are allowed to help choose, for example, the pictures to be displayed, there is a markedly higher level of commitment to the results and a reduction in the level of damage and general deterioration. Patients and staff have commended the commitment and skills of all of the interior designers commissioned by the SHSA, and welcomed their own involvement in the process. Papers by Brian Chapman and Ruth Preece in *The*

Arts in Health Care: A Palette of Possibilities (Kaye and Blee 1996) describe the direct involvement of patients in arts projects at Ashworth Hospital.

LANDSCAPING

The benefits of good design are not restricted to buildings. Each of the Special Hospitals provides quite literally acres of scope for landscaping and the integration of buildings with their surroundings. It is the landscape which brings parts of the hospital together in a coherent whole, providing a sense of order and clarity and enhancing the quality of life. It makes a significant contribution to the perception of visitors and neighbours and can do much to soften the custodial imagery of the large Special Hospital sites.

The SHSA recognised the importance of landscaping for each of the Special Hospitals. Ashworth Hospital in particular has been the subject of considerable landscaping development in recent years. The flat, north site is bounded by a high wall which obstructs views over local countryside. For patients here the wall is the horizon, perhaps for many years. It was natural then to focus landscaping measures here. One aim of the Development Control Plan for relocating services from the south site was to ensure that all of the space between buildings should be planned, interesting and cared for. Here landscaping is more than simply decoration; it integrates the buildings and forms a series of articulated and contained spaces within the hospital. Blocks of planting have been introduced which divide the site into a series of groups of wards, or neighbourhoods.

Because of the lack of views from that part of the site, one aim has been to create internal views from features of interest, including items of modern sculpture. Trees have been planted around the internal perimeter which, from a distance, screen the wall and create the illusion of space which continues beyond the perimeter – without compromising security.

On the east site, the new Jade and Amber wards were designed from the outset so that buildings and grounds are complementary. Here the site is flat, featureless and bleak. The aim has been to create gardens which serve as a continuum of the indoor spaces and to give the impression of private gardens to one side of the ward and a larger ward garden for group use on the other, providing patients with a choice of privacy or activity.

The above gives some insight into the contribution made by landscaping. An article by John Lynch in *The Arts in Health Care: A Palette of Possibilities* (Kaye and Blee 1996) provides further insight into its application to hospital sites and more detail of his work at Ashworth Hospital.

PREVENTION OF SELF-INJURY AND SUICIDE

Self-injury and suicide attempts are regrettably a feature of life in psychiatric hospitals and pose a real challenge for those designing and managing them. The challenge in design terms is to create an environment which reduces the potential for self-harm and suicide to a minimum whilst remaining attractive, stimulating and not overtly custodial. Measures which make the acts of self-harm and suicide as difficult as is reasonably possible need to be incorporated into a setting which appears relaxed and patient-friendly and which promotes the treatment and rehabilitation processes. They should not result in a bleak, in-stitutional, alienating setting, but should result in a sense of the normal.

In March 1995, following pioneering work in this area by Broadmoor Hos-pital and co-ordinated by John Lynch, the SHSA published a design guide on this specialist area: *Suicide Preventative Measures: Design Guidelines and Checklist* (SHSA 1995). The Guide addressed both direct design measures and contribu-tory measures which need to be taken into account within the framework of a suicide prevention strategy. It acknowledges that provision of a 'normalised' environment carries with it an element of risk which needs to be managed, but stresses that layout and planning of wards and individual rooms should assist staff in managing these risks, going on to provide examples of good practice and design drawn from the experience of a wide range of hospital staff over many years. The concluding section of the guide provides a very detailed checklist of potential risks and appropriate preventative measures.

PERIMETER SECURITY

The creation of a more therapeutic built environment went hand in hand with a substantial programme of investment at each of the hospitals to strengthen and upgrade the perimeter envelope – the system of walls and electronic measures installed to secure the perimeter. With a strong perimeter barrier in place, the regime within the secure area and the secure envelope of individual buildings can be less restrictive, with direct benefit in terms of patient behaviour and treatment. Whilst it has proven costly and difficult to introduce these physical changes to the perimeter which effectively open up the interior of the site, changes in attitudes and practices will now be needed if this new potential to liberalise is to be exploited to the full. In 1996, following work by John Lynch and others, the SHSA codified and published its own standards of physical se-curity.

CENTRALISATION VERSUS DECENTRALISATION

Tensions between these two aspects of site development emerged throughout the seven years of the SHSA's redevelopment of the hospital sites. Central provision of facilities for visiting, dining, recreation, rehabilitation and sport – an institutional characteristic – offers advantage of economies in construction and staffing – though it does entail a great deal of escorted patient movement. By contrast, decentralised, ward-based or perhaps locally-based facilities are expensive to provide, involving an element of duplication in construction and not benefiting from economies of scale in staffing. But they are valuable in delivering a more personalised, less institutional service. A balance needs to be struck. Provision of locality-based sports facilities is clearly uneconomic but provision of, for example, facilities which permit patients to receive visitors on the ward is entirely practical and is a welcome and far cry from the familiar mass visiting sessions in the hospital central hall. The development of locally-based clinical team bases, each serving a local group of wards, as adopted during the reconfiguration of Ashworth Hospital, provides benefits in terms of improved accessibility and in the relationship between the clinical team and its patients.

SYSTEM BUILDING

This was employed by the SHSA, working in close collaboration with Ashworth Hospital, to adopt a completely fresh approach in the construction of the new Jade and Amber wards on the hospital's east site. The aim in constructing these wards was to provide a rapid response to the need to close the south site (for reasons of greater integration and economy), whilst providing modern, attractive buildings which met fully both the SHSA's environment standards and those set out in the SHSA's Ward Design Guide in an economic manner. Essentially this involved design and construction of both wards and adjacent landscaping *de novo* within a year and within a budget of £2.2 million – substantially cheaper than anything which had gone before, challenging conventions with regard to speed, cost and design principles. These aims were achieved by adopting a systems build approach, whereby many of the components are constructed off-site and assembled on site. But more fundamentally, their design involved a re-examination of the principle whereby every ward needed to be constructed to the highest standards of robustness.

Historically, Special Hospital wards have been designed to accommodate the most challenging patients, challenging in terms of their propensity to abscond and to inflict damage to themselves or to the ward. In the traditional secure ward, all patients live in an environment designed to withstand the most challenging. The resulting building is overly restrictive and forbidding for the majority but carries the advantage of being entirely flexible with regard to the types of patient who can occupy it. Buildings designed on this basis are expensive.

An alternative approach is to design the new building with a particular group of patients in mind – in the case of Amber and Jade wards, two target

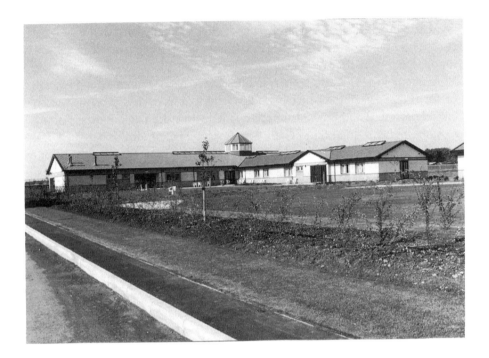

Figure 8.2 Amber Ward, Ashworth Hospital

groups – the elderly and those patients being prepared for discharge. This approach permitted the design of a building which was less repressive, less obviously 'secure' and with a more domestic ambience. It permitted the adoption of less heavyweight construction methods and a systems-build approach, with resultant saving in time and money. Many of the building components were constructed in a factory in Scotland, transported and assembled on site.

The buildings, which are located in a purpose-landscaped area, are of single storey, brick-clad construction. They feature wide windows which are glazed with shatter-resistant polycarbonate plastic which obviates the need for bars. The large panes create a light and airy feeling and provide an unimpeded view of the grounds whilst maintaining a high level of security. The interiors comply with the SHSA's standards: wide corridors lead off a central living area which has been designed with high ceilings, a central lantern and roof-lights to maximise the amount of daylight entering the building. Décor was selected by patients and staff working in collaboration with interior designers who co-ordinated the overall design. Furniture is as attractive as possible whilst retaining the necessary features of safety and durability. Observation panels to patients' rooms, traditionally just slots, have been designed as an integral part of the doors and each patient has access to personal en suite facilities.

One evident advantage of the quick-build approach was, as described above, the involvement of staff and patients, who would go on to live and work in the building, in the detailed design process. During the course of design of these wards a 'mock-up' patient's room was constructed and installed on site for viewing by staff. Aspects of its design were modified as a result of staff comments.

UPDATING THE PHYSICAL ENVIRONMENT – VALUE FOR MONEY?

During the SHSA's seven-year existence, capital of the order of £100 million was invested in the three Special Hospitals. Of course a proportion of this was for the normal run of replacing and updating time-expired services (water, drainage, electrical supply, heating etc.), but the greater part was invested in providing a better standard of life and improved treatment facilities for the hospitals' patients – some of the country's most serious and dangerous offenders. Can it be justified? What was achieved? Was it worth it? Could not the money have been better spent?

The case for investment on this scale is rooted firmly in the fact that the residents of the Special Hospitals are patients and not prisoners. The special hospitals exist to treat, not to punish, and in common with other NHS patients, their patients have a right to decent, supportive living conditions which promote rather than frustrate their treatment and rehabilitation. This case is particularly strong given that their length of stay in hospital is amongst the longest of all NHS patients, averaging about seven years.

Any future programme for the relocation of Special Hospital patients to other sites would inevitably be a long-term, protracted task. It was therefore the SHSA's aim to provide acceptable standards of accommodation on the three existing sites. The improvements described do just that, improving the quality of life, treatment and prospects for some of society's most unloved and unlovable.

THE APPLICABILITY OF THE LESSONS LEARNED

A number of aspects of the SHSA's work may have wider application. The following are offered for consideration:

- o Development of patient-centred environmental standards appropriate to the organisations aims; audit of existing buildings and construction of a prioritised, remedial development programme. This has significant potential application to facilities for the elderly, learning disabled and mentally ill in all forms of institutional setting.

o Regular (annual) review and reporting of progress made in moving towards these standards.

o The importance of formally and regularly reviewing standards and design guidance so that they remain relevant and credible.

o An examination of the case for alternative design solutions (e.g. systems building) and procurement routes (e.g. design and build), perhaps employed in concert.

o Adoption of a policy which ensures that professional interior designers are engaged not only on new-build schemes, but on all refurbishment projects. Their involvement should be from the outset, not as an afterthought.

o The opportunity for patients to participate in the design process and, in particular, interior design and the selection of pictures and other decoration.

o The integration of building design and landscaping; the conscious setting aside of funds for the latter as an integral part of building development.

o A careful consideration of the concept of risk management in relation to the design of secure buildings; a consideration of the implications of 'over security' for patient behaviour and treatment. A presumption that overt aspects of secure design will be kept to a minimum consistent with safety and manageable risk.

REFERENCES

Kaye, C. and Blee, T. (eds) (1997) *The Arts in Health Care: A Palette of Possibilities*. London: Jessica Kingsley Publishers.

SHSA, London (1992) *SHSA Ward Design Guide*. London: Special Hospitals Service Authority.

SHSA, London (1995) *Suicide Preventative Measures: Design Guidelines and Checklist*. London: Special Hospitals Service Authority.

CHAPTER 9

Industrial Relations

Charles Kaye and Alan Franey

THE AUTHORITY'S EXPERIENCE

The Starting Point

Industrial relations in the Special Hospitals at the time of the SHSA's arrival could be likened to a country suffering from rampant inflation. Those nominally in charge were directed by forces below them to courses of action which only seemed to feed what they wanted to cure.

Senior managers in the hospitals felt no real authority in dealing with their staff. The Prison Officers' Association had an enormous membership among virtually all types of staff (amounting to between 70 per cent and 80 per cent of the total employed). No other union had a significant presence and the Department of Health met only with the POA for negotiations and consultation, thus neatly bypassing local (hospital) management. That management had the will to challenge the POA's domination but after bad experiences (such as at Moss Side in 1988) felt that they would not be backed by the Department in a crisis. The suspension of staff by management for infringing hospital rules provoked a retaliatory 'locking up' of patients by the POA and, in the face of this action, the Department surrendered to the POA's demands, revoking the suspension. Managers felt abandoned. Soon after that they were actually made redundant by the Department to pave the way for the new Authority!

The POA dominated each hospital in terms of which practices were acceptable: either in the clinical sphere (where the threat of 'security' was used to oppose all manner of changes); or in the personnel sphere where restrictive policies were rigidly maintained (such as a 'promotion' policy which was a 'dead man's shoes' approach which favoured existing staff and militated against outsiders).

The union did have the virtue of defending its members, usually in situations where no other body supported them. But such defence was virtually indiscriminate: the closing of brotherly ranks in the face of any threat to any individual. Underneath the formal carapace of the union, unwholesome behaviour thrived with threats and intimidation being regularly deployed against any individuals who dared to oppose the prevailing union culture. The Ashworth 'dirty tricks' Inquiry in 1992/93 provided ample evidence of this.

The inbredness of the hospital reinforced this brotherhood: many staff lived on the hospital estate, took their leisure in the hospital social club and had spouses and/or other relatives working alongside them. In such a hothouse, the luxuriant growth of an aggressive and obdurate union overshadowed more delicate growths.

With new management, at the centre and in each hospital, conflict was inevitable – but not sought.

Management's Approach

We needed to be fair and consistent. We moved forward with the following principles:

1. To be available for, and to encourage, discussion, consultation and negotiation with the unions.

2. To support all health service unions within the hospitals, urging them to expand their membership and representation.

3. To define key policies, in discussion with, but not subject to the veto of, the unions.

4. To ensure that we communicated directly and frequently with our staff and did not regard the union as the only, or even the key, channel for that.

5. To keep the Department of Health out of any direct dealings with the unions. Thus we had to convince the Department of the wisdom of this course of action and help them restrain their addictive impulses to dabble in detail.

6. To maintain a united front, Authority and managers, to ensure we were not divided, centre from hospital, hospital from hospital, and picked off.

In practical terms, these principles translated into a series of actions spread over some years. This is now history recollected in tranquillity; then it was sweaty and uncomfortable work in the face of the forge where well-banked fires blazed.

Key Actions

We created a central bargaining body – a joint consultative and negotiating committee – where *all* unions were represented and where staff side membership was calibrated to prevent the POA from swamping the proceedings completely. The emergence of RCN and UNISON representatives as chairman and secretary of the staff side added enormously to its effectiveness.

We were painstaking in defining which matters were for consultation and which for negotiation. In the event of deadlock over consultation we could, and did, use the Authority itself to adjudicate on key issues affecting staff.

Although we did meet unions individually at HQ level on occasion, we tried to avoid that, not least because meetings with the POA were so depressingly predictable. A long opening harangue – often from John Bartell, their then National Chairman – would accuse management of a range of perfidious behaviour that Machiavelli himself would have admired. After this 'softening up', a range of outrageous demands would be made. Once these sterile proceedings had closed, a POA emissary with a white hat would sneak round the corner offering to intercede and tone down the demands! How unprofitable, and how wearing. Probably the most sensible discussion with the POA took place at hospital level, although the bullyboys also played at that level.

We produced a range of key policies to demonstrate management's concern for the staff, to define boundaries and offer a constructive partnership binding staff and management. So, policies on sickness and absence from work, training and study leave, staff welfare and counselling, disputes and grievances, discipline and appeals were all taken through the consultation process and implemented. All the time these policies were shared directly with staff at the hospitals so that they understood what was happening as management saw it.

This process was studded with disagreement but also, slowly, illuminated by mutual understanding about the need for policies to exist – and to be honoured by all.

Within the management ranks we worked hard to ensure that we were united, thrashing out our own differences in private and keeping in close touch with developments in each hospital.

Challenges

Besides the everyday pressures which could focus on such elementary but important features as the escorting of patients (where the POA pursued its inflationary bent, calling for multiple escorts in almost every circumstance), we anticipated a major challenge. When we approached the abolition of the assisted travel scheme for staff, we realised it had the potential for explosion. The special hospitals alone, in all the NHS, retained this anachronistic device which paid staff part of the costs of travelling to and from work. It was frankly an unjustifiable 'extra' and we proposed very reasonable phasing-out terms which the POA would not accept and which were subsequently imposed.

Shortly before Christmas 1990 the POA started industrial action at Ashworth Hospital using the device of manning levels for escorting patients. This was in response to the dispute about the travel scheme payments and was quickly escalated once management refused to roll over. The POA called an all-out strike on the wards at both Ashworth and Rampton Hospitals. Broadmoor Hospital had only token action since they had only one member of staff remaining on their travel scheme. Virtually all the nurses at the first two hospitals withdrew their labour, leaving nurse managers, other professional staff and administrative and clerical staff to man the wards. And this they did – for nearly a week despite all the pressures and dangers and – at Rampton – the additional hazards of a severe blizzard and a subsequent power cut.

The Department of Health were obviously concerned but allowed the SHSA to pursue its course. A face-saving agreement – which conceded nothing – was agreed and the staff returned to work. From management's point of view, we had seen the worst – and survived. At hospital level, many managers and professionals got new insight into patient care and new evidence about unacceptable practices. From the POA's point of view, they had deployed their heavy artillery but failed. Their action caused much bitterness, between staff and between staff and patients. The SHSA, by a majority, agreed to report all trained nurses who had taken strike action to the UKCC and although that case was eventually rejected, the seriousness of their situation shocked many nurses. Thereafter, POA influence and membership began to decline – although both are still significant in today's hospitals.

At about the same time we lost ground in another exercise. The national re-grading of nursing staff was taking place and we agreed to a joint exercise with the Department. The result was overgrading throughout the hospitals, a reflection of the familiar device of 'buying your way out'. As nearly always this was the wrong approach and did not remove problems but only postponed their appearance on management's agenda. A year later we would have had the confidence to be firmer.

Similarly, we never got to grips with the Special Hospital Lead and Environmental Allowance. These were – and are – payments made to most of the hospitals' staff, originally as a device for recruiting and retaining them. In total it amounted to several million pounds for which management received nothing. It did not help us find the right staff but it did tend to keep existing staff, producing an unhealthily low turnover reinforcing a lot of the negatives already described. Towards the end of the SHSA's life, we started to chip away at the allowance with a view to converting it to a performance-linked system of payments but we ran out of time, passing the system, and our aspirations, on to the new Hospital Authorities.

We had set up an appeal machinery within the disciplinary procedure. After progressing through managerial levels an independent tribunal was included – chaired by an SHSA member sitting with two other individuals drawn from a panel agreed by the Joint Consultative Committee. Naturally unions used this machinery to challenge managers' decisions: and sometimes the panel over-threw the decisions. This always caused great distress to the managers who found it difficult to accept that an appeal process was not there just to support management. It did sharply remind managers of the need to conduct and pre-pare disciplinary action thoroughly.

Devolution

Our goal always was, once key policies had been agreed, to focus industrial re-lations and communications at hospital level. That was the epicentre of activity where contact between staff and management would be most frequent and should be most profitable. As the hospitals developed their own personnel (later human resource) departments this transfer of responsibility became more of a reality. The need for unity on key issues remained and we used the SHSA's managerial network to ensure that unity was maintained.

With the recognition that the three hospitals were destined to become inde-pendent Authorities in their own right, we accelerated the process of devolu-tion. Most significantly we dissolved the central negotiating and consultation machinery and set up local equivalents at hospital level. This was strongly con-tested by all the unions – who saw it as a divorce from the centre of power – but to us it seemed an inevitable and proper step.

As a result of this carefully orchestrated programme of policies and devolu-tion, we left each hospital well equipped for the management of staff within the new Authority. What a pity those Authorities didn't start – as we recommended – by derecognising the POA!

A HOSPITAL'S EXPERIENCE

Many people will recall the turbulent relationships between employers and em-ployees throughout the Public Sector in the 1960s and later with 'the winter of discontent' in 1979 which ultimately led to the downfall of the then Labour Government and saw Mrs Margaret Thatcher arrive at 10 Downing Street. In the years that followed there was still industrial unrest and during the mid-1980s there was the long-running miners' dispute in Nottinghamshire and Yorkshire which led to many pit closures and an end to the mining industry as we had known it over the years. During that turbulent period there was a good deal of peer pressure on miners who were members of the National Union of Mine Workers; this pressure was about conforming and supporting industrial action and those who, for whatever reason, expressed the wish to work would find their families in small mining communities isolated by colleagues and property damaged. I recall witnessing bitter scenes between families on television and even to this day disharmony still remains in what is left of the mining communities.

In October 1988 I first visited Broadmoor Hospital as part of a task-force which had been put in place by the Department of Health following the highly damaging Health Advisory Service Report. When I arrived there was industrial action ongoing between the Hospital Managers, Department of Health and the Prison Officers' Association which at that time had sole negotiating rights within the hospital despite rising membership in other organisations. Staff morale was low and the reasons for this are complex. Discontent was reflected in the content and quality of debate and negotiation between the POA and Managers which appeared more concerned with conditions of service than innovation or therapeutic advances. Suspicion and rumour tended to proliferate. The HAS Report recommended that staff organisations should consider the constructive role that they could play in improving patient care by different ways of working. 'Red rag to a bull', said one employee.

One of my first tasks was to negotiate with the Prison Officers' Association in an attempt to reach a settlement of the dispute. There was a general lack of co-operation between the key players which amongst many things led to a hospital building for over 100 patients, newly furbished at a cost of £30 million, being left empty for a long period of time. The Prison Officers' Association were not prepared to co-operate with management in discussing the commissioning of the new building. It was a quite scandalous situation.

The task-force which included unusually Sir James Savile OBE, who had been associated with the hospital for many years, realised that in the months ahead we would face a turbulent period, and consideration was given to the possibility of seeking Ministers' support to bring the army into the hospital. The hospital had relied very heavily on the use of overtime and on those occasions where nurses refused to work overtime the hospital was virtually brought to a standstill which sometimes led to patients being confined to their rooms. Several discussions were held with senior officials at the Department of Health and Ministry of Defence at the same time as discussions were continuing with the Prison Officers' Association in an effort to bring about an end to the dispute. After a short time the dispute was resolved, however, it was clear to me that any attempt to introduce radical change as demanded by the Health Advisory Service Report, which said that time was running out for the hospital, was going to be met with fierce opposition.

As time went on it became clear to me that there were similarities between what had happened within the mining industry and what happened in the Broadmoor Hospital community. A community which included staff houses, hostels, the hospital itself and a staff social club which played its role as the hotbed for the POA. There were well-motivated employees who were very keen to introduce change; however, this met with a fierce reaction from some of the hard-liners who saw their role as looking after criminals rather than patients with mental health problems. For those that did not conform there was damage to their personal property, that is, their cars and homes, and in the local Crowthorne community verbal aggression in supermarkets by families of staff. It made me more determined to grasp the nettle and bring about change.

Following the establishment of the Special Hospital Service Authority (SHSA) a National Joint Consultative Committee (JCC) was set up with representatives of all recognised trade unions meeting with the Authority's Executive Directors and each of the General Managers from the three Special Hospitals. This was mirrored by the establishment of Joint Consultative Committees at each of the hospitals. One of the difficulties encountered in introducing these new arrangements was the unwillingness at first of the POA to sit at a table with other recognised trade unions. The POA had long been the sole union with negotiating rights and the SHSA were determined that other trade unions who had members working in special hospitals would be recognised. After the initial difficulties and squabbles over the new arrangements the POA finally agreed to participate as managers made it quite clear that if they did not then they would be excluded from any consultation or negotiation. There followed arguments about how many representatives from each recognised trade union would sit on the Joint Consultative Committee and who would chair the staff side of the committee. There was a fundamental problem in attempting to bring about change and that was the stance taken by the Prison Officers' Association who deemded that special hospitals should not be part of the National Health Service but run as part of the Prison Service; that still remains their view today.

I was surprised at some of the existing procedures that had been negotiated primarily with the POA for dealing with disciplinary matters, and one of the first tasks of the JCC was to consult and negotiate a revised procedure. After a great deal of debate this was achieved although the POA refused to accept the new procedure. Despite that it was introduced. A range of other procedures and policies including a Facilities Agreement and a Grievance Procedure were produced. As a member of the National JCC it was interesting to witness the power-play between the RCN, NUPE, COHSE and the POA and quite often it was more a case of hot air than real meaningful discussion. I was relieved when the SHSA took the decision to disband the National Committee and devolve all negotiation and consultation to each of the three hospitals.

In the early 1990s there were major conflicts between the POA and each of the three hospitals which led to strikes by POA members at Ashworth and at Rampton Hospitals although fortunately not at Broadmoor Hospital. A good deal of pressure was put on the local POA officials to take some form of action and this amounted to patients being locked in their rooms for five hours before management could negotiate an end to this unauthorised seclusion. The Branch Secretary of the local POA at that time played a very significant role in bringing about this settlement and I was extremely grateful to her. There were of course casualties as a result of this unauthorised seclusion and whilst the POA enjoyed the bullyboy tactics of exerting its authority it found itself in a much weaker position when patients' representatives reported qualified nurses to the UKCC. These qualified staff had the dilemma of either unlocking doors and then facing the backlash of other colleagues as I mentioned earlier in this chapter or keeping the doors locked and finding themselves in breach of their Code of Conduct. There are still nurses at the hospital today who have a blemish on their record imposed by the UKCC. It became clear that the Prison Officers' Association did not fully understand the role of nurses and the differences between prison officers in the Prison Service and the responsibilities of nurses in a Special Hospital. Much of the progress that followed industrial action depended largely on who was leading the Prison Officers' Association at the hospital. We went through periods of considerable difficulties with one particular Chairman who had his own agenda and I believed that leaks to the media about patients, particularly those with a high profile, were not just coincidental. During the early 1990s it was necessary to move a number of staff out of the hospital as I was clear that progress would not be made with some of the individuals who had hardened attitudes towards change. Staff welfare was important and new arrangements were introduced to provide counselling services for the staff. What was important for me was to find a way to communicate directly with staff rather than rely on staff associations. I set up a communication network with representatives from different parts of the hospital who would meet at frequent intervals to be given briefings by managers and as you would expect this left some trade union officials and managers feeling uncomfortable. I nevertheless was determined that there would be more direct communication with staff. As part of this change I introduced 'The Hot Seat' which were open meetings not only for myself but also for senior managers at the hospital and members of the SHSA who would be available for hourly sessions for any member of staff to come and quiz on any issue that was concerning them within the hospital. This approach proved quite successful and I had many sessions with some very lively debate.

As has been said elsewhere in this book the Prison Officers' Association is effective and from its members' perspective it represents them well, particularly in the Prison Service. However, the POA is still diametrically opposed to Special Hospitals being part of the NHS and this can be seen from the vigorous campaign that they ran in conjunction with a national newspaper in 1997 which led to the then Secretary of State, Steven Dorrell, setting up a review of services at Broadmoor Hospital. This in my opinion was quite unnecessary and showed political weakness. It is now, though, time to consider the very question of recognising a Prison Service union in a Health Service environment. Broadmoor Hospital became a statutory authority in its own right in 1996 and the question of whether the POA should be recognised was discussed at the highest level; the advice received was that from a political point of view the timing was not quite right given that a general election was looming in the months ahead. Perhaps another example of political weakness. The Special Hospitals are often seen by the public as part of the prison system and this is reinforced when the POA representatives are discussing matters with the media. The very fact that it is a representative of the Prison Officers' Association continues to give the wrong impression to the outside world. There is no doubt that if the Special Hospitals are to change then the prison culture has to be removed and in my view the Prison Officers' Association should no longer be recognised. This Association is not recognised in the NHS Whitley negotiating machinery and plays no part in other health establishments. It is important for those committed staff who wish to see real change and who enjoy working in the special hospitals to be represented by associations that have a genuine interest in health care and not in a deep-rooted culture and a controlling environment.

I feel pleased with the progress that has been made but there is still a long way to go.

PART 3

Focusing on the Patient

CHAPTER 10

Describing the Patients

Margaret Orr

SPECIAL HOSPITAL PATIENTS

The individuals treated in Special Hospitals must fulfil two basic criteria. First, they must be detainable under the terms of the 1983 Mental Health Act (MHA). Second, their behaviour or offence must be deemed sufficiently dangerous to pose such an unacceptable risk to the general population (either individually or *en masse*) that detention in lesser security is unsafe. However it is hoped that a description of some important issues will help the understanding of the patients treated in our 'special places', although these criteria encompass a wide range of background factors impossible to elaborate on in this chapter.

A new, if somewhat clumsy word has been coined by some professionals looking at the factors contributing to mental disorder. It is 'bio-psycho-social'. For our patients, 'bio' would have to encompass congenital abnormality, birth injury, childhood and teenage trauma and accident, epilepsy, brain damage caused by drug and alcohol abuse, the brain damaging effects of mental illness itself and side effects of medication. 'Psycho' would have to cover cognitive discrepancies, that is, false concepts derived from upbringing or development, abuse in childhood, be it physical, emotional or sexual, trauma from childhood or adolescent loss and parental separation or deficiency in adult role models.

'Social' would mean damaged families, frequent moves in early life, criminality and educational misfits resulting in poor qualifications and unemployment. In other words, 'bio-psycho-social' for the Special Hospital patient covers a vast range of difficulty and of course there are exceptions. Some patients are admitted from what appears to be a 'normal' background and it is their overwhelming disease which has resulted in the dangerous behaviour. More often however it is a complexity of background factors and a diffuse range of damage such that the resultant 'treatment' has to tackle an intricate and fluctuating state of disease. To complicate these issues there are also political overtones often related to the offence itself: Health Service disputes as authorities debate funding for discharge; and Home Office, including Parole Board, involvement and public concerns. Permeating this, the patient has a personal need to come to terms with the guilt, remorse and responsibility for the behaviour. In broad terms this 'spiritual' or 'philosophical' need, whether or not it is related to a God, is at the heart of therapy, creating a whole person with improved self-esteem awareness and responsibility. These patients are inevitably difficult to manage, challenging and complex in their treatment. The following paragraphs may be useful in giving a flavour of this.

THE ROLE OF THE SPECIAL HOSPITAL

There is the unpalatable reality that society requires to send to a Special Hospital those who have so hurt and offended the sensibilities of that society that nothing less than maximum confinement and restriction will do. The Special Hospitals become the repositories of the fears, anger and pain of the nation they serve. The patients have often been the scapegoats in their own families, schools and societies. They have frequently reacted with aggression to their situation or perceived situation. Our role is not to condone or forgive, that is for their God and their victims, but to aid their understanding and render them less ill or diseased and hopefully make them safer to return to society.

The task of the hospitals is to find the meaning of the dangerous behaviour for the patient, for the health professional and for the public. This understanding is of paramount consideration for the Mental Health Review Tribunals (MHRT) and the Home Office, who control the transfer or discharge of restricted patients, and is also important for the consultant psychiatrists and tribunals who consider the non-restricted patients.

This understanding must become apparent in terms of knowing the circumstances concerning the onset of the behaviour, the nature of the mental disorder, the contribution of drugs or alcohol, the social, family and emotional life of the person prior to the violent or dangerous act. The patient also needs to know the nature of his or her own mental disorder, the interaction of that disorder with other social stressors, the need for and response to medication, supervision and monitoring. Probably the most difficult aspect, for patient and carer, is the balancing of acknowledgement of responsibility, victim empathy, guilt, remorse and debt to society against the need to instil self-esteem, confidence, integrity, awareness and hope for the future. Before admission, the less understanding there is of the patients and their behaviour the more likelihood there is that they will be sent to a Special Hospital and the longer they will stay. It has always been the task of the Special Hospitals to promote this understanding but they have been aided since 1989 by the establishment of management accountability, increased openness to external scrutiny and, from the patient's

Ten Tribunal Tips

1. Mention you played cricket at Boarding School.

2. Tell the Judge you'll vote Tory if they drop your Section!

3. Say you feel you are a drain on NHS resources by staying here.

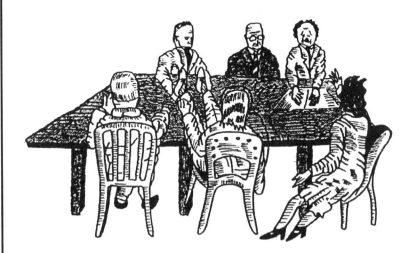

4. Repeat continually 'Broadmoor has been the best thing that's ever happened to me.'

5. When your RMO says you are a danger to yourself and others and you are personally responsible for the Iran–Iraq war, the fall of sterling on the world stock market, Euro-football problems, you must agree with him/her.

6. Respectfully mention that you have spent 43 years in Special Hospitals.

7. *Never ever* raise your voice/boot/fist, in anger.

8. Turn your Walkman down when they directly ask you questions.

9. If it is a lady judge compliment her on the superb wig she's wearing.

10. Always say thank you at the end, even if it's been a disaster.

Figure 10.1 'Ten Tribunal Tips' from the Broadmoor patients' Chronicle

point of view, increased awareness of their needs and a more varied range of therapeutic options in line with the rest of the National Health Service.

MHA CLASSIFICATION/DIAGNOSIS

To fulfil the first criterion for admission we first consider the two main legal classifications of the 1983 MHA under which patients are detained in Broadmoor Hospital: the psychopathically disordered and the mentally ill.

THE PSYCHOPATHICALLY DISORDERED

Although comprising just over a quarter of all admissions to Special Hospitals, the group with the legal category of psychopathic disorder (PD) are often regarded as most contentious. Special Hospitals provide the only secure treatment facility, outside prison, where compulsory admission over longer than two years is needed. It seems illogical to presume that the current time-limited Medium Secure Units could seek to change in two years those who by the very definition of their disorder have exhibited dangerous behaviour and a disordered personality for many years. In the past some Medium Secure Units would manage those with personality disorder both as inpatients and outpatients, using medication at times of profound affective or mood change and at times of psychotic breakdown (i.e. separation from reality), but as pressure on beds increases so it has become rarer to find such units which will accept PDs showing anything but transient dangerousness. It has been left to a few wards in the Special Hospitals to take on the unenviable task of treating those whom many regard as untreatable but who are clearly in need of help.

The security risks experienced in trying to treat those who are devious, dangerous, and often skilled in criminal activity, in institutions primarily geared to looking after the mentally ill are all too evident (as at Ashworth in 1996 and 1997). Most PDs who are eventually admitted have been tried for treatment on an interim hospital order (MHA, Section 38) for its maximum term of six months (three months renewed monthly until six months) but this still occasionally fails to tease out those reluctant to continue their commitment to therapy once the hospital order with or without restriction (MHA, Section 37/41) has been granted. Several show great interest in individual and group dynamic psychotherapy, the cognitive behaviour and 'social' therapies offered along with the creative therapies (art, music and drama) during their six-month assessment period, but when in-depth therapy starts and the inevitable pain of maturation, acceptance of responsibility and growth begin to bite, the patient may cease to participate in a meaningful way.

It was possible for intelligent, charming individuals to appear to be keen for therapy during their six-month assessment but, once the hospital order was imposed, to 'back off', adopting a conforming complying stance, taking part in physical work activities but failing to tackle the underlying emotional/psychological work. They could spend years being the perfect patient, con their way through MHRT and re-enter society only to reoffend, even with psychiatric and social supervision. Fortunately there is hope that these cases are becoming fewer as the most rigorous of admission assessments is conducted (Bailey and MacCullough 1992). With the development of more research by the new Professorial Units, established by the SHSA in the Special Hospitals, and a finer sifting procedure at admission it is hoped that only the most appropriate will be offered treatment and that the treatment will be more focused on patient need.

The deviousness of those with psychopathic personality disorder makes them exceedingly difficult to treat and it is for this reason that many experienced forensic psychiatrists opt for the manoeuvre of offering treatment in hospital following sentence by the court, that is, transfer from prison to hospital (Section 47/49) during sentence. To others it seems unacceptable to form the opinion that someone is mentally disordered, in need of treatment and yet to send them to prison. For the friends and relatives of the victim and for the teams involved in looking after these patients, disastrous outcomes cause long-felt distress and heartache. Fortunate and mature is the forensic team who come to terms with the reoffending of their former patients.

The type of personality disordered patient who appears most amenable to treatment within Broadmoor Hospital seems to be the person who has had an associated degree of affective disorder present at the time of the offending or dangerous behaviour, who has been dependent or anxious and perhaps with a degree of paranoid personality disorder. By using the medication for the active symptoms and techniques to improve self-awareness, self-esteem and confidence with realistic goals and objectives; by gradually increasing the degree of responsibility by challenging cognitions and providing an increasing range of choice and tasks (e.g. keys to their lockers and rooms, free access to gardens, with education and tasks related to capability) combined with insight therapy both individual and group; and by taking into consideration the abuse which many of the patients have been subjected to, it has been possible to aid the maturation and rehabilitation of some of them.

It is rare indeed to find a patient in Broadmoor with a legal classification of psychopathic disorder who has not been abused in childhood either emotionally, physically or sexually. Although it is in the women patients that the degree of sexual abuse in childhood has been most frequently remarked upon, a significant proportion of male patients have also experienced abuse. It is the degree of the abuse, the way in which it was revealed, and other factors in the child's environment, such as schooling, attentive adult or the existence of physical illness, which contribute to the way in which the abuse is exhibited. For example, a young man with schizophrenia, undiagnosed till his third prison sentence for raping his mother, did not reveal his being forced into male prostitution from the age of eight until he had been three years in Broadmoor and was in group therapy. Until then he had been regarded as a very aggressive psychotic patient who attacked others without reason. Knowledge of his abuse helped the team to make sense of his delusions (false beliefs held against reasoned argument and outside one's cultural experience).

The Professorial Unit at Broadmoor, opened in 1995, runs a ward which is primarily focused on the therapy of the psychopathically disordered but it is seen as important to apply the skills learned in looking after those with personality disorders to help the mentally ill. Psychological treatments are essential for both groups and many would say there is little difference between the two groups apart from the use of medication for the mentally ill.

THE MENTALLY ILL

Three quarters of the patient population are detained with a mental illness (MI) and, for the vast majority, the illness is schizophrenia.

It is here we need to consider the debate about the mixing of mentally ill patients with those considered to have a primary diagnosis of personality disorder. Usually patients with mental illness have been treated elsewhere before coming to a Special Hospital although this is by no means universal. However in most the illness has been difficult to ameliorate and in many there have been detrimental effects on the patient's personality as a result of their illness. This may cause diminished ability to express feelings, loss of pleasure in life, poor ability to make friends or socialise, insensitivity to social norms, difficulty in communication, with stereotyped thinking, odd mannerisms and appearance resulting in isolation in a hospital ward.

Our patients have often acted on their delusions or responded to their hallucinations. One of the treatment aims is to clarify: why this patient? why this delusion? why now? The woman who sought to kill all Pakistani pharmacists was subject to prosecution by one after she stole from his shop. Superficially her delusion that all Pakistanis are bad was based on that experience but as knowledge of her increased so we discovered cruelty by a Pakistani grandmother in her teenage years after prolonged deprivation by her own mother. Self-image and self-esteem destroyed from childhood take time to rebuild by using both practical and psychological therapies and it has been in linking these that advances have been made over the past few years. Sometimes the illness has been present for so long that a preponderance of so-called negative features of schizophrenia appears with passivity and lack of initiative, poor self-care, marked apathy, aimlessness and a total social withdrawal. The old workshops (tailor, carpenter, leather work, radio repair) of the Special Hospitals aimed to tackle these latter problems but there was little identification of individual need. Unfortunately this type of facility is expensive to run and is endangered by current funding as they are not economical for small numbers.

Those with active schizophrenia will often respond to their auditory hallucinations and may act on them in anti-social ways, such as exposing themselves or urinating in public, or becoming physically aggressive. The combination of people with mental illness and those with personality disorders on the same ward can result in flash points of violence as the ward gradually comes to terms with how to function satisfactorily. But there can also be advantages as the PD learns tolerance and responsibility and the schizophrenic patient is stimulated to converse and interact.

BEHAVIOURAL REASONS FOR ADMISSION

Thus disorders of personality and mental illness are the 'medical' reasons for admission but what are the dangerous behaviours which result in admission? There are some types of behaviour which raise the possibility of admission. Actions such as the targeting of a specific victim and persistence in contacting the victim either by stalking, attacking or threatening will be likely to cause alarm. One such example is the case of the man who wrote three letters to three victims. In the first he told his victim he would kill her on a Thursday, in the second he said he would kill his victim at work and the third victim was told he would first kill her daughter then her. The first victim stopped going out on Thursdays, the second gave up her job and the third moved away. The escalating nature of the violence described in the letters had ever increasing effects on the victims. However the violence may not be aimed at an individual but at a class or group, such as the woman who wishes to kill male babies, writing in blood to maternity hospitals and new mothers, or the man who wants to kill all black young men or another who wants to attack women in authority. In these latter examples, the generalised nature of their victims makes them difficult to manage in lesser security than a Special Hospital as it is impossible to protect this wide range of victims. Escalation of violence from expressing the violent thought through repeating with vehemence a delusion, such as believing you will be the saviour of womankind by killing all women who wear trousers, to following women, to carrying a weapon, to attacking a woman by punching, or to stabbing a victim, obviously raises the likelihood of admission. Acting out even in a trivial way on delusional beliefs is a sinister progression as is the carrying out of commands given by auditory hallucinations. Recent work in the United States (Monahan and Steadman 1994) reveals that it is the feeling of being under the control of an external force or person which is a dangerous prognostic sign in patients suffering from schizophrenia, and we are finding the same evidence here.

Although roughly one third of patients who come to a Special Hospital have not been convicted of a crime, nevertheless their behaviour has been considered to be too dangerous for management in any other setting. One woman has a conviction for a minor offence of going equipped to commit criminal damage. She was arrested in the grounds of a hospital equipped to break in. She had previously tried to suffocate her mother, pursued two female doctors by phone call, letter and visits, made threats to kill another female psychiatrist (and continues to do so), attacked a policewoman, broken into a psychiatric clinic to destroy her notes, and confessed to the arson of a £140,000 rehabilitation unit but was not convicted. Since admission she has attacked a female forensic psychiatrist, has walked along a 14ft wall (internal) in Broadmoor, persecuted a male psychiatrist in the hospital and made weapons from curtain rails. Despite this she presents well at her annual MHRT and an argument is always made that she has only minor convictions against her name. She continues to be detained due to her mental illness and behaviour and not because of her 'index' offence.

Fire is by far the most common reason for women to be admitted to Broadmoor. Frequently it is in the context of self-harm but it may be simply the pleasure of watching things burn or the satisfaction of revenge. Another method of assault which is taken seriously is poisoning as the serious poisoner, particularly the mentally ill poisoner, often retains his or her knowledge of poisons and has a ready but secret weapon to hand. One man with a developmental condition called Asperger's Syndrome has a profound knowledge of medical toxicology and delights in rhyming off various household goods which he could use to poison someone if he wished. This is said, not with any malice, but in the sheer pleasure of carrying out an experiment. He is otherwise the most charming, helpful and earnest of men but clearly requires a degree of external control on his behaviour.

Although patients cannot be admitted solely because they exhibit sexual perversion or sexual offending, nevertheless many Special Hospital patients have committed a sexual offence – perhaps linked to some of the histories as mentioned above. Anger against the opposite sex due to real or perceived ill treatment combined with the anger from fear of personal violation, loss or rejection may culminate in a sexual offence or the acting out of a delusional state in a disorganised sexual attack. The Special Hospitals fulfil a useful purpose in treating those who exhibit mental disorder, either MI or PD, combined with sexual offending as the ability to treat in a unisex dimension initially is helpful with later controlled therapy with the opposite sex where issues of victim and perpetrator may be worked through. There has been much criticism by women's action groups of the 'use' of women as guinea pigs to test out the men's progress in therapy in these psychotherapy groups but to stop this would be to deny the women the chance to express their own feelings about being victims and to prevent the ultimate in therapy which is to accept responsibility for one's own action and understand how one arrived there. However, the therapists need to be experienced and sensitive to prevent scapegoating, further victimisation and escalation of psychopathology, and it is difficult to ensure that group confidentiality is not breached.

The most common offence for men patients, and the second most common for women patients, is homicide but on average our patients spend longer on a hospital order than they would do if they received a life sentence for manslaughter. As in all cases of homicide, the victim is most often known to the patient, perhaps a member of his or her own family or an intimate social contact. At other times the conflict and anger within the family setting may be projected onto an acquaintance or the person may be involved in the 'crossfire' as a bystander. The mentally disordered most frequently do not plan. Naturally there are exceptions, such as the paranoid person who carefully plots and schemes how to retaliate against perceived oppression or persecution. Despite these facts there remains great fear in the public's perception that our patients are somehow going to be released to cause mayhem.

Much of the work done in hospital is in helping the patient come to terms with their offence, for example going over the depositions and hopefully allowing them to develop a sense of responsibility without tipping them over the edge of a guilt-ridden suicide. This latter possibility is a constant concern for the therapist working with this vulnerable group.

TREATMENT

There are practical elements in the treatment of patients. Drug and alcohol abuse prior to admission is so common in our patients that it is worthwhile screening / assessing all. Taking cannabis may have few serious consequences for the average person, but for those with a predisposition for mental illness, those with mental handicap and those with underlying personality disorder it can be disastrous and often is. For example, the girl who regularly took cannabis failed to act on her auditory hallucinations until she combined cannabis with alcohol and amphetamines. As she swung from the top of a crane throwing paint tins down at police, she literally felt on top of the world. She developed a complex paranoid delusional system involving a female psychiatrist of whom she had only a vague acquaintance, put the doctor's life at risk and is now in a Special Hospital. It appears to the patient in hospital that their addiction problems have gone; some of the men and most of the women become dependent instead on prescribed medication, drinking Diet Coke by the two-litre bottle, demanding their 'prn' (per res necessitation), that is, medication given as required, or cutting themselves in an addictive way. These are not pejorative statements but a recognition of the serious dependency needs of these damaged people. They have no inner 'good parent', no ego strength and no self-esteem.

All they have is their immediate pain and they want that relieved now! Treatment is directed at helping them recognise situations which cause anger, helping them build up an inner comforter in the therapeutic relationship, developing other more productive coping skills through communication and helping them tackle their anxiety and anger. In order to address the problems of forensic addiction a new unit was opened in Broadmoor in 1995 with the support of the SHSA.

Many of the patients have concomitant physical or organic damage either from congenital conditions or caused by birth injury or trauma in childhood. They may have injuries in adolescence or damage by alcohol / drug abuse. This may be minor and only show on a brain scan but it is the combination of minor deficit and mental illness and/or personality disorder which compounds the picture and renders therapy complex. Learning about cooking, budgeting, domestic cleaning, laundry and personal care are all ways of developing the patients' skills, developing self-esteem and overcoming problems. All aid socialisation and confidence and form an important strand in therapy.

There is a complex interaction with the outside world in the form of relatives, friends, solicitors, voluntary agencies, Mental Health Act Commission, probation, social work, victims and victims' families and an equally complicated network in the hospital world of nursing staff, medical staff, social workers, psychologists, psychotherapists, occupational therapists, creative therapists, educational staff, administration staff, hospital management and last, but by no means least, other patients. This creates a vast network of communication, emotional upheaval, information and misinformation, social and psychological pressure, support and destructive power, sexual involvement, memories, sympathy, criticism, confusion and occasionally help.

The patient is at the centre of this vast range of competing and supporting forces and has to adjust to the hierarchy of power on the ward both in terms of pecking order of other patients and the staffing structure of the ward. He or she must learn whom to trust and who is influential. They need to know who is dangerous and they often have anxieties about previous acquaintances, either from prison, if they have been convicted of a crime, or from another hospital where their behaviour may have been problematic. Past behavioural 'baggage' is frequently embarrassing and the patient wants to be in control of their own information. Yet they come into a system where control is removed from the beginning.

THE FUTURE

For the future it remains essential to preserve a range of therapies within secure settings to address the varied and complex therapeutic needs of the patients. These are people who are deemed to have had their responsibility for their actions reduced by their mental disorder. The quality of life of these patients must be preserved if we are to call ourselves a humane society. Locking them away for life to guarantee the public safety would promote hopeless warehouses of people with demoralised staff and patients alike. Thankfully there is now hope for a modern forward-thinking series of institutions based on the underlying tenets of the SHSA for a high quality of investigation and treatment, based on patient need and measured by improved health and lessened dangerousness. This is perhaps still uncomfortably closer to hope than actuality but at least the requirement has been identified and accepted by most of us who work within Special Hospitals.

REFERENCES

Bailey, J. and MacCullough, M. (1992) 'Patterns of reconviction in patients discharged directly to the community from a Special Hospital.' *Journal of Forensic Psychiatry 1013*, 445–461.

Monahan, J. and Steadman, H.J. (eds) (1994) *Violence and Mental Disorder (Developments in Risk Assessment)*. Chicago: University of Chicago Press.

CHAPTER 11

Learning Disability in the Special Hospitals

Diana Dickens

INTRODUCTION

Special Hospitals have a long history of catering for patients with a learning disability. The population is concentrated in two sites, namely Ashworth Hospital and Rampton Hospital.

Fashions have changed in admission patterns to Special Hospitals and up to 20 years ago it was normal to admit both children and also people who were not a public danger in the true sense of the word. In the last 20 years, however, it has been conceded that special hospital placement, in many cases, is no longer appropriate for people with a learning disability.

In 1972 the Butler Report stated that in the development of medium secure facilities there was no place for patients with severe learning disabilities (SLD) who should be catered for in their own specialised service. Medium secure units should however provide for people with mild learning disabilities (MLD). In practice this did not take place. In the past this created pressures on Special Hospitals to admit people in this category even if they were not a 'grave and immediate danger' because their management in other situations caused serious problems. Latterly, however, admission criteria for this group have been rigidly enforced.

Equally there were still cases of people with SLD who posed a severe risk to carers but whom it was still felt reasonable to admit to Special Hospitals. As an indication of the intractability of SLD cases, their average length of stay in Special Hospitals is 18 years as opposed to a norm of 7–8 years.

THE CLIENT GROUP

People with learning disabilities have a level of intelligence which is under two standard deviations below the mean of normal distribution curve of intelligence. This is estimated to equate with an IQ of approximately 70. Further sub-divisions are made so that there are categories of MLD and SLD.

All patients within the special hospital system who suffer from learning disability will be detained in Mental Health Act terms of mild mental impairment or severe mental impairment. The definition of severe mental impairment incorporates the term 'severe impairment of intelligence and social functioning in association with abnormally aggressive or seriously irresponsible behaviour and that detention is necessary for the health and safety of the patient or the protection of other persons'. In addition, with mental impairment where the degree of impairment and social functioning does not amount to severe impairment it is stated 'that it is appropriate for the patient to be treated in hospital and that such treatment will alleviate or prevent a deterioration of the patient's condition'. In the definition of severe mental impairment it is stated that patients will require care and supervision so that they are not a danger to themselves or other people.

The legal system establishes a differentiation into two groups, such divisions being reinforced by other factors:

1. Genetic

It is generally accepted that genetic influences and abnormalities account for a high percentage of people in the group with SLD, whereas people with MLD form the lower end of a normal curve of distribution of intelligence levels within the general population.

2. Butler Report

This report differentiated between MLD and SLD in terms of provision of secure facilities (see above).

3. Behaviour Patterns

People with SLD tend to exhibit challenging behaviours, that is, injury to care staff and a spectrum of other anti-social behaviours which make their care extremely difficult (stripping, smearing of faeces, self-mutilation and severe damage to property). However, it is unusual for this group to reach secure services via the courts as people with such a degree of disability are not usually charged. Therefore most special hospital patients in this group are cared for under Section 3 of the Mental Health Act.

People with MLD, however, frequently present through the courts and are detained in special hospitals under the categories of Section 37 or 37/41 (restriction order). Although the offences occur across the whole spectrum of offending behaviour it is generally recognised that offending levels occur in relation to arson and sexual offences with an incidence above that in the normal population.

OTHER CONDITIONS ASSOCIATED WITH LEARNING DISABILITY

Mental Illness

Mental illness within people with a learning disability is increased in incidence and its manifestations can vary from those of the general population. Various studies have indicated that learning disability is associated with a higher than normal incidence of offending behaviour and that low IQ is a crimogenic factor in its own right (West 1982).

Prevalence figures in the many studies range from 8 per cent to 15 per cent of the population with learning disabilities with serious disorders, but with the inclusion of minor disorders the incidence may rise to over 50 per cent (Fraser and Nolan 1994).

In SLD it is unusual to make a formal diagnosis of mental illness in view of the absence of speech and general level of functioning.

With MLD, although speech content can be simplified, it is often possible to describe paranoid ideation plus hallucinatory and delusional systems. Also in this group patients who are particularly prone to depression can often describe their reactions to life events which have caused them to lapse into such a condition. Anxiety states occur too which can range from generalised anxiety states and agoraphobia to specific phobias.

Epilepsy

Overall in people with learning disability epilepsy is extremely common (up to 50 per cent of people). Its aetiology is variable and may range from birth injury to genetic defects, for example tuberose sclerosis. Its incidence increases with the degree of learning disability.

Sensory Defects

Sensory defects are another source of handicap which can contribute significantly towards the manifestations of learning disability, for example auditory and visual impairment.

Autism

Autism is a very common concurrent condition with learning disability, 75 per cent of people with autism falling within the SLD category. Although not all these people have full-blown autism many people with learning disabilities have autistic spectrum disorders, not amounting to the full autistic complex, which cause difficulty in management and which underlie many of the most serious and intractable considerations (Wing 1994).

These factors demonstrate that the population within the Special Hospitals suffering from learning disability has general characteristics which are different from people within the range of normal intelligence. Medicine has acknowledged this fact in the creation of a specialist qualification for learning disability nurses (RNMH) and also in psychiatry where consultants have a special training in learning disability which recognises the very special needs of the group as a whole and also the different characteristics of MLD and SLD.

The above factors indicate that not only should the learning disabilities population have a specialist service which is separate from mental illness provision but also that MLD and SLD require different management strategies.

TRENDS IN THE MANAGEMENT OF LEARNING DISABILITIES OUTSIDE THE SPECIAL HOSPITALS

The 20 years prior to the SHSA's formation had seen huge changes in learning disability services within the community, starting with *Better Services for the Mentally Handicapped* (DHSS and the Welsh Office 1971). This recognised that people with learning disabilities require to be cared for with equal rights to other members of the population, and initiated the move away from large learning disability hospitals to smaller community homes. Care in the community was seen as a way of achieving these ends but also saving money by the closure of large old-fashioned mental handicap hospitals. However in recent years it has been accepted that community care can be a more expensive option if sufficient staff are provided to give an appropriate standard of care and treatment.

Although the move took place gradually there was a transfer of psychiatric services into the community (for example, the provision of community psychiatric nurses) and many consultants, contracts reflected the need for time to be spent in the community as well as the hospital.

By the end of the SHSA's reign most of the learning disability hospitals had been closed and the majority of patients were enjoying a more normalised life in community placements such as small group homes, hostels and also increasingly by staying at home with parents rather than being admitted to institutional care.

SPECIAL HOSPITALS AND CHANGES IN GENERAL PHILOSOPHY

Until the late 1970s, the populations in both Moss Side (as it was then) and Rampton Hospitals remained relatively static in number as it was very difficult to get services to take back patients with a history of Special Hospital admission. Whilst it was accepted that the old learning disability hospitals cared for many people with very challenging and difficult behaviours, authorities who were looking to close these down did not relish with enthusiasm having to fund very expensive placements for this group of people. It was not possible for special hospitals to provide a 'dowry' and in addition to this, catchment areas did not have to pay for special hospital care.

Therefore, there were perverse incentives to prevent the discharge of people from the Special Hospitals. However, following the Boynton Report (1980) on Rampton Hospital it was recognised that there were considerable numbers of people with a learning disability who were trapped in the system, and at Rampton at least there was a large impetus to try and discharge people from the special hospital service. Patients were discharged due to huge effort and a change of emphasis in rehabilitation for people with a learning disability. This change was also recognised at Moss Side, although there was not perhaps such an impetus at that time.

LEARNING DISABILITIES AND THE SHSA

The Formation of Ashworth

When the SHSA came into being in 1989 the majority of learning disability patients were in Rampton Hospital and Moss Side Hospital, the latter specialising mainly in learning disabilities. Moss Side and Park Lane merged almost immediately after the SHSA came into being to create Ashworth Hospital.

Should Services be Provided at Broadmoor?

Rampton and Ashworth hospitals divided a catchment area of England, Wales and Northern Ireland between them. Therefore many patients were cared for far from their place of origin.

Following the reign of the Office Committee of the Department of Health and Social Security who managed the Special Hospitals, the SHSA had a unique opportunity to arrange for the provision of a unified service for learning disabilities to serve the entire catchment area. This, however, highlighted the question of whether a learning disability service should be developed in Broadmoor to enable the population of the south of England to have a more locally based service.

Table 11.1 Learning disability patients: referrals, admissions and departments 1988–96

All hospital referrals		Ashworth		Rampton		Broadmoor		All hospitals	
		Adm.	Dep.	Adm	Dep.	Adm.	Dep.	Adm.	Dep.
1988	41	5	13	11	21	-	1	16	35
1989	42	8	6	4	11	-	1	12	18
1990	30	6	7	4	10	-	-	10	17
1991	24	5	11	5	10	-	-	10	21
1992	21	2	8	3	12	-	-	5	20
1993	19	1	9	4	20	-	-	5	29
1994	17	-	8	2	16	-	-	2	24
1995	20	-	4	4	15	-	1	4	20
1996	n/a	-	9	3	11	-	-	3	20
Total	214	27	75	40	126	0	3	67	204

In October 1990 the SHSA convened a workshop to debate how the services of the Special Hospitals should develop. The group considering learning disabilities decided, after vigorous discussion, that a service, in theory at least, should be developed at Broadmoor and to serve this end a feasibility study should be conducted. As a result of this, negotiations took place with the Academic Department of Psychiatry at St George's Hospital, London, for the establishment of a joint post at Senior Lecturer level between themselves and Broadmoor during the next 18 months. Unfortunately it was not possible to attract a suitable applicant for the post.

Surveys of Special Hospital Patients

It was decided by the SHSA that in order to estimate quickly the special hospital population in terms of security needs a survey should be conducted of all Special Hospital patients on one day in March 1991. Although it was agreed that this was only a rough indication of security needs, it was of particular interest in that it differentiated between security as supplied by purely physical means (perimeter security) and that provided by high staffing levels, careful observation and management and security procedures (internal security). These factors were estimated as both perimeter and internal security were assessed for each patient (in a total population of 256).

This survey attracted the attention of the *Guardian* who proclaimed that 'Only 50 per cent of Special Hospitals patients needed to be there'. It was possible to obtain mental impairment and severe mental impairment figures separately. This showed that only approximately 25 per cent of learning disabled patients required maximum security, which equated with a level of security provided by Special Hospitals (Table 11.2).

Table 11.2 Survey No. 256: Patients rated separately for internal security and perimeter security

	Medium security or less		Maximum security		Total
	Perimeter	Internal	Perimeter	Internal	
Mental impairment	120	39	60	147	366
Severe mental impairment	68	26	8	44	146
Total	188	65	68	191	512

Table 11.2 indicates that: there is a population of SLD requiring maximum security, but this is residual in nature and since 1990 following the SHSA's decision not to admit any more patients with SLD there have been no further admissions; there is a considerable need for MLD maximum security.

The question of patients' needs for treatment and security was further quantified in 1993 by Maden *et al.* (1995) who carried out a 20 per cent sample of the special hospital patient population. Amongst other things the research esti-

Table 11.3 Patients with a secondary diagnosis of learning disbilities: estimated security needs now (1993) and in 5 years

	1993		1998	
	N	%	N	%
Maximum security	21	29	13	18
Medium security	27	38	21	29
Local hospital locked ward	11	15	12	17
Local hospital open ward	7	10	8	11
Community	6	8	18	25
Total	72	100	72	100

Source: adapted from Maden *et al.* (1995)

mated the current and future security needs of the patients with learning disabilities who were sampled. The results of which are presented in Table 11.3. Allowing for extrapolation of the 20 per cent this would show that a sizeable number of people (approximately 100) needed conditions under maximum security in 1993 but the estimation was that by 1998 this would be reduced to approximately 65. This ties in with SHSA statistics which indicate that by the end of the century the number of people requiring maximum security will fall to about 50 or 60.

The Formation of the Learning Disability Steering Group

In 1992 it was decided to form a steering group, chaired by the Chief Executive of the SHSA and including general managers of the hospitals, which looked at the development of a unified service to meet the needs of the patients with learning disabilities.

By this time, at Ashworth an audit had been undertaken of all Special Hospital patients with learning disabilities who could be cared for in less secure environments. Fifty per cent of the existing population could be moved on and with a corresponding reduction of admission rates a dramatic decline of patient numbers was anticipated. A social worker was appointed who was given the specific responsibility of leading a project to achieve the rehabilitation of patients with learning disabilities.

At Broadmoor it was agreed that there was a continuing need for a small team led by a senior nurse to come forward with proposals for future development. At Rampton, due to continued action in rehabilitation of patients with learning disabilities, the patient population was declining rapidly and it was agreed that an audit as at Ashworth should be undertaken.

It was also of note that the Mentally Disordered Offenders Report on Services for People with Learning Disabilities (mental handicap) and with Autism (Reed 1994) had been published and three strands were picked out for consideration by the group – research, staffing issues and autism.

SHSA STRATEGY FOR DEVELOPMENT OF SERVICES FOR PATIENTS WITH LEARNING DISABILITIES

Discussion Paper

A discussion paper was produced by the SHSA, the main thrust of which was to evaluate the Broadmoor development. In the consideration of the decline in patient numbers it quoted from the Gunn/Maden report: 'for the 30–40 per cent of cases which needed maximum security it was impossible to imagine that they would obtain a similar standard of care and quality of life in any other setting'.

It also contained the advice that the 'Purchaser/provider market might impinge on the Special Hospitals in that they might become independent Trusts'. This would impact on the learning disability services in as much as there would

Table 11.4 Admission trends in all hospitals from January to December 1990–1992 inclusive

		1990	1991	1992	Totals	
					Referred	Admitted
Ashworth	Ref.	10	5	11	26	
	Adm.	5	2	1		8
Broadmoor	Ref.	0	1	1	2	
	Adm.	0	0	1		1
Rampton	Ref.	22	11	14	47	
	Adm.	6	4	8		18
Total					**75**	**27**

Source: Ashworth documents.

be pressure on the service to avoid reduplication. The question posed by the strategy was: should a single site be developed in Rampton as there may not be enough demand for all sites?

Admission Trends: Work Commissioned by the SHSA

Clearly the reduction of patient numbers in the Special Hospitals depended not only on the rate of discharge of patients but also on the admission rate. The admission rate is also important because if the assumption is made that the admission criteria are being correctly applied it reflects the true level of future need for special hospital places.

It shows that,in general there was a reduction of admissions with the exception of Rampton in 1992 and also that a considerable number of referrals were made which were not accepted.

At Rampton a survey was done from July 1990 to June 1993 of admissions of learning disability consultants' patients which showed that there was a total of 19 admissions detained as mental impairment during this period. Sixteen patients were admitted once and three patients were admitted twice.

Three patients had dual diagnosis of PD/mental impairment and two patients had dual diagnosis of MI (mental illness)/mental impairment. It should be noted:

- No severe mental impairment.

○ Five non offenders.

○ Fourteen offenders including one patient detained under Section 35 and subsequently Section 38.

It can be seen that the figures in Table 11.5 represent a concrete need for the future to detain patients with mental impairment in conditions of maximum security.

Table 11.5 Classification of admissions to Rampton Hospital July 1990–June 1993

Section	No.	
Sec. 3	4	Non-Offenders
CPIA	1	Non-Offenders
Sec. 35	4	For Assessment Offenders
Sec. 38	1	For Assessment and Treatment Offenders
Sec. 37	3	Hospital Order Offenders
Sec. 37/41	6	Hospital Order and Restriction Order Offenders
Sec. 47/49	1	Transfer from Prison Offenders

Note 1: CPIA = Criminal Procedures (Insanity) Act.

Broadmoor Service Proposal

In May 1994 Broadmoor Hospital presented their service proposals for a Learning Disability Service. A team had been assembled which identified 41 patients, who were from the southern catchment area, suitable for relocation in the south, 28 patients in Rampton, nine in Ashworth and four in Broadmoor.

Four service proposals were made but already by this time anxieties were being expressed about the viability of setting up and resourcing a new facility when it had been amply demonstrated that the population of Special Hospital learning disability patients was declining. The projections showed a population of 50–65 by the year 2000 and the SHSA decided that in view of these facts the project at Broadmoor should be abandoned.

The SHSA and Service Specification

In order to reflect movement to the purchaser/provider ethos at the end of 1993 the Steering Group started to work on a service specification which engendered much debate. The fourth draft emerged in July 1994. It defined the scope of the service as being for people with MLD and seriously violent or challenging behaviour. Treatment provisions should be comprehensive with the aim of returning patients to their own communities. Other points made were in general line with existing practice. There should be a comprehensive range of treatments, and where the patient was not recommended for admission the clinical team would continue liaison work with the referring agency as appropriate. With specific reference to the provider it was stated that the provider would develop appropriate measures which would enable others to judge its performance in achieving its declared aims.

An outline of baseline service planning for 1994/5 requirements and statement of 1995/6 requirements of patients with learning disabilities were significant. It was also stated that detailed costs should be prepared for 1995/96. It was suggested that proposal contracts should initially be block contract with each provider based on occupied beds. The SHSA would commission the purchase of these bids. A service specification was produced.

The Final Year of SHSA

Although sharpened by the purchasing arrangement for 1995–96 which it was anticipated would 'shadow' for new purchasing arrangements, the prospect that in April 1996 the Special Hospitals would become autonomous SHAs directly accountable to the NHS executive, took attention away from strategy at a national level. However this was redressed by the publication of 'Service Strategies for Secure Care'.

Service Strategies for Secure Care

At the end of 1995 the SHSA produced a document entitled 'Service Strategies for Secure Care'. A chapter in this document talked about strategy for patients with learning disabilities. The contribution of the Maden survey (Maden *et al.* 1995) was recognised and some of the broader issues other than the purely numerical were acknowledged. For example, Maden found that patients with learning disabilities in hospital had a range of other psychiatric problems and that their perceived therapeutic needs were not dissimilar from the needs of other patients with mental illness, that is, the full panoply of multidisciplinary care and psychological and psychiatric treatments.

A comment was made that for the 30–40 per cent of cases rated as needing 'maximum security' it was impossible to imagine that they could obtain a similar standard of care and quality of life in any other setting. The ability of Special Hospital nurses to manage many of these patients with only occasional use of seclusion was noted as was the range of occupational therapies. It was the team's impression that these patients enjoyed a better quality of life in a Special Hospital than they would elsewhere.

Although the Mansell report (1993) wished to close the old 'mental handicap hospitals' as quickly as is practicable, it was considered that the special characteristics of those patients with learning disabilities who are considered to be in need of high security must be born in mind. This guidance to the National

Health Service makes it clear that those who need additional treatment for psychiatric illness or severe behaviour disturbance may require specialist treatment in hospital settings.

The strategy summarised the argument to support the development of a National Superspecialist Service based on a single site. As the NHS is developing an increasing number of locally based medium secure beds for patients with learning disabilities the Special Hospital population will continue to diminish. The advantages of developing such a single-site service would be to focus expertise and develop a super speciality within the high security service, cultivating a broad range of knowledge and skills among staff who provide care and treatment to this difficult group of patients. Also such a concentration of resources could be more cost-effective than a dispersed service.

In the document the Board of the SHSA considered that two principles needed to be followed in the provision of this service. Firstly, it should not replicate what exists elsewhere and, secondly, patients who do not need high security care should not be cared for in the Special Hospitals. The report concluded that in view of the diminishing number of patients at Ashworth Hospital and the lack of learning disability beds in Broadmoor, the best way forward for the future was to focus on the development of a single-site learning disability service at Rampton Hospital.

CONCLUSION

The past decade has seen the closure of many old and large learning disability hospitals. However, even in the population of these hospitals there is a hard core of people who require specialist nursing, medical and other interventions for the treatment of their challenging behaviours. There has been a concern in learning disability services that this closure of institutions has led to a 'de--skilling' of RMNH nursing staff who are less able to cope with severely challenging behaviour. There is now a feeling in the development of community services generally that there is a need for specialist services for those with challenging behaviour, mental illness and those who offend, which has to be provided by the Health Service (Day 1994).

It is acknowledged that the staff at Rampton Hospital have a long history of being able to treat and manage well and humanely the population of patients with learning disability which the hospital contains. This not only includes medical and nursing treatment but also the facilities such as the Occupational Therapy Centre (Rosedale) where a wide variety of occupational, social skills and other educational needs are met. It is also very important that this group of patients have 'space' (Wing 1994) which the Rampton campus provides. There is a concern that were this group of patients to be dispersed all this expertise would be lost.

Following the strategy statement in 1995 that Rampton should continue to develop its specialist national service for learning disability there has been further agonising over the future of Special Hospitals. Murphy (1997) in a recent editorial is quoted as saying that there is no reason to prevent the closure of the Special Hospitals and that in fact this should be encouraged. Against such categoric assertions the future for learning disability may have to be reviewed. If this situation were to arise it would appear that a learning disability service could be the most vulnerable for early relocation.

Nonetheless it has to be accepted that in the future there will be an ongoing need for maximum security. Patients with mild learning disabilities have demonstrated their ability to overcome very robust perimeter security and in the present political climate the need to protect the public is high on the agenda.

It would still seem, using the statistics quoted earlier, that a nationally specialised service should be continued and, in view of the case already made, that were the special hospitals to close, this care could be continued in a purpose-built unit of approximately 50 beds. If this were to be the scenario it is important that some of the mistakes made in the closure of the old learning disability hospitals should not be repeated, namely attempts to cut costs and the dissipation of a highly skilled and motivated work force.

REFERENCES

Boynton Report (1980) *Report of the Review of Rampton Hospital* (Cmnd 8073). London: HMSO.

Butler Committee, The (1972) *Report of the Committee on Mentally Abnormal Offenders*. (Cmnd 6224) HMSO.

Day, K. (1994) 'Psychiatric services in mental retardation – genetics or specialised provision?' *Psychiatric Disorders in Mental Retardation*. Cambridge: Cambridge University Press.

Department of Health (1993) *Services for People with Learning Disabilities & Challenging Behaviours or Mental Health Needs*. London: HMSO.

DHSS and the Welsh Office (1971) *Better Services for the Mentally Handicapped* (Cmnd 4683). London: HMSO.

Fraser, W. and Nolan, M. (1994) 'Psychiatric disorders in mental health retardation.' In Bouras (ed) *Mental Health in Mental Retardation*. Cambridge: Cambridge University Press.

Gunn, J., Maden, A. and Swinton, M. (19) 'Treatment needs of prisoners with psychiatric disorders' *British Medical Journal 303,* 338–41.

Maden, A., Curle, C., Meux, C., Burrows, S. and Gunn, J. (1995) *Treatment and Security Needs of Special Hospital Patients*. Whurr Publishers.

Murphy, E. (1997) 'The future of Britains high security hospitals.' (Editorial) *BMJ* No. 7090, 3 May.

Reed (1994) 'Review of Health and Social Services for Mentally Disordered Offenders and others requiring similar services' Vol.7. *People with Learning Disabilities (Mental Handicap) or with Autism*. London: HMSO.

West, D.J. (1982) *Delinquency, its Roots Carers and Prospects*. London: Heinemann.

Wing, L. (1994) 'The autistic continuum Chapter 1D psychiatric disorder in mental retardation.' In Bouras (ed) *Mental Health in Mental Retardation*. Cambridge: Cambridge University Press.

CHAPTER 12

Patients as Intimate Partners
Resolving a Policy Crisis
Pamela Taylor

DIFFERENTIAL ATTITUDES TO RELATIONSHIPS

Whenever people are together, friendships and enmities will develop between them, and romantic and sexual relationships will occur. Nobody regards this as remarkable in ordinary society, in which the vast majority of people consider themselves healthy and free to choose partners. The pleasures of such relationships are highly valued in all sorts of ways, including the emotional warmth and support, physical intimacy and the giving or reinforcement of self-worth that they bring. The challenge of maintaining such relationships or the pain of splitting up when they go wrong are also recognised, but scarcely amount to an overriding consideration in the heady days of making one.

Ordinary people may, in fact, not have as wide a choice as they believe. Society perhaps regulates the relationships of its members more than is generally acknowledged. If the observational and management skills described in Edith Wharton's novel *The Age of Innocence* (1920)now seem less impressive and oppressive, and arranged marriages are prevalent in some cultures only, even in western society the family remains a form of institution and still seeks some influence on the pair bonding of its members. Wider society tends to support this with explicit laws, unwritten rules and, often unsolicited, opinion.

People who are seriously and chronically ill or disabled, or in some other kind of trouble, may perceive no less a need for romance and sex, but, if their healthy or relatively law-abiding peers notice, then they are commonly puzzled, even repelled or censorious. If the sick or troubled are brought together in some kind of society specifically made for them – perhaps a hospital, a hostel, a prison – then those healthy peers become more definite in their restrictive views and in any case the nature of the 'made' society is such that it carries its own regulations which will limit social fulfilment within that setting. The rules may be explicit and well founded; after all many people who are chronically ill or disabled, and many offenders too, are very vulnerable and open to exploitation. More often than not, however, there is no explicit guidance for staff or residents, no open discussion of the issues, and covert practices evolve which lead to avoidance of recognition of relationships where possible and destruction or heavy limitation of any that break through. Such 'management' by default can be as dangerous as it is inhumane.

A CHANGE IN THE LAW ON MARRIAGE: A REVIEW OF POLICY

The Special Hospitals, the home at any one time of about 1600 people who have serious chronic mental disorders and have, generally as a consequence, also behaved very dangerously in some way, were prompted to emerge from this sort of chaos by the recognition by a few patients that the law no longer saw them as unfit for marriage. Article 12 of the European Convention asserts a right to marry and have a family that must be accorded to all of marriageable age; it acknowledges only some specific limitations in national laws such as consanguinity or pre-existing marriage. Test cases have established the rights of UK prisoners to marry (*Hamer; Draper*). While the rights of people compulsorily detained in hospital on the grounds of mental disorder have not been tested in case law in the UK, it is considered that the only limiting factor might rest in their capacity to make contract – in this case a contract of marriage. All that is required is that the person must be 'capable of appreciating that it involves the responsibilities normally attaching to marriage' (*Park*). The level of appreciation is regarded as 'basic', that is so simple that it is hardly likely to be possible that it could be impaired.

Lawyers advised that an objection on grounds of mental disorder to the marriage even of a patient resident in a Special Hospital would be likely to be regarded by the Court as 'frivolous'. A small number of marriages took place. The law does not, however, further support conjugal rights; the European Court ruled that the denial of conjugal association to husband and wife held within a secure institution was 'no violation' of Article 12; Article 8, which guarantees a general right to privacy and family life, allows that those rights may be restricted for 'the prevention of disorder or crime' (*X and Y*). Other formal rights do, however, follow from legal status – including that of recognition as 'nearest relative' under UK mental health legislation, and, with this status, the right to challenge the partner's detention and be a party to detention review hearings. (For a further discussion of the legal position see Fitzgerald and Harbour in press.)

In the early 1990s, no recognised hospital or social facility could be identified in England or Wales which was prepared to rehabilitate as a couple patients who had married in special hospital and become ready for discharge. Other romantic and potentially sexual relationships emerged without the backing of formal contract. Similarly no recognised facility or professional body was able to supply a working policy or procedure for assessing or managing marriage or other such relationships within an institutional setting. It was necessary to devise them.

SPECIAL HOSPITAL PATIENTS:
A FOCUS FOR EXPLICIT POLICY

A Special Hospital setting is the best of places and the worst of places from which to contemplate a risk – benefit analysis of relationships between couples in regulated communities, and strategies for their assessment, management and treatment. Much of the possible variance is there, to extremes. The partner/patient-centred problems are greater than almost anywhere else: the institution is closed and secure, with all the special problems that that brings for staff and patients alike; there is particularly close scrutiny by lawyers of the activities therein – and thus of rights as far as they go; and the mass media cannot resist a prurient interest in anything to do with sex given that the population includes one or two nationally, even internationally, notorious cases in which deviant sex and violence have been prominent.

In reality Special Hospital patients are suffering from some of the most serious mental disorders. About two thirds of the men and half of the women have schizophrenia; about one quarter of the men and one third of the women have a severe personality disorder, within the legal classification of psychopathic disorder; and most of the remaining small group have a behaviour disorder in conjunction with mental retardation or severe retardation (Taylor et al.1998). Two thirds of the men and 80 per cent of the women have a history of childhood loss of a parent or similar disruption (Ferraro et al. in press); preliminary figures suggest up to 80 per cent of the women and just over 50 per cent of the men have suffered *prolonged* physical abuse, sexual abuse or both. Over 90 per cent of the 1500 or so men and 75 per cent of the 300 or so women resident in any one year have been convicted of a grave criminal offence, about two thirds homicide or other serious personal violence, 15–20 per cent arson or firesetting and around 10 per cent of the men explicit sexual offences; among the technical non-offenders a similar range of behaviours short of homicide had triggered admission. All are compulsorily detained. The average length of stay for men with a mental illness or personality disorder is about 7.5 years, for women around 10 years, and longer for people with one of the mental retardations. In a real sense, then, the hospitals become their home; postponement of response to relationship needs until an acute illness has subsided and the patient has returned to the community is rarely a serious solution. To what extent should rights to relationships be protected?"What demand is there anyway? To what extent do rights to safety and health compete? Is staff intervention of some kind inevitable?

ATTEMPTS TO STUDY RELATIONSHIPS

Other people's relationships in any circumstances appear to constitute a difficult, even neglected area of enquiry, particularly when those relationships include sex. Serious attempts to study them meet with derision. The USA national survey of the early 1990s (Laumann *et al.* 1994), for example, met with a barrage of criticism of social science methodology in general and self-report in particular. One of the principal problems for the scientist is that there are some things that occur within a couple that cannot be directly observed, because to interpose an observer would, by definition, destroy the dyad. For the critic, however, there appears to be an assumption that if the members of the couple are asked to report what goes on between them, they will necessarily want to distort the truth. Lewontin (1995), a leading geneticist, was one such critic. He singled out the finding that 45 per cent of the men between 80 and 85 reported having sex with their partner as so patently untrue that, without the need to provide any contrary *evidence*, the validity of the whole survey could be called into question. In fact, the contended finding was compatible with evidence from a handful of other studies of relationships and sexuality more specifically targeted at older people (e.g. Pfeiffer *et al.* 1969; Mulligan and Moss 1991). Similar kinds of denial of sexuality have extended to psychiatric patients, others with chronic illness or disabilities and others who are institutionalised.

Duggan (in press) explains the neglect of formal assessment of couples in clinical practice in part in terms of the general neglect of couples therapy among the psychotherapies. He suggests that this is firstly because of the challenge of integrating a number of different types of psychotherapy in the single approach and secondly because of the perceived difficulty in trying to understand two individuals simultaneously rather than one alone. Of the latter he points out that Skynner (1980), a family therapist, argues that in individual work it is much more difficult to avoid being manipulated, or placed in the role of judge, supporter or persecutor rather than therapist. A balanced, realistic approach to work which impinges on relationships is more likely to emerge from work with the couple.

In psychiatry more generally, concepts of pathology are also almost invariably centred on the individual. In very unusual circumstances a disorder incorporating more than one person is given a name, such as when two or more closely related people share a psychosis – *folie à deux*; more commonly there is no such formal recognition. It is perhaps partly why so many clinicians are uncomfortable with the assessment and treatment of people with a personality disorder. Almost every category recognised in the International Classification of Diseases (WHO 1992) incorporates in its definition some disability in close relationship formation or maintenance. The Committee on the Family, Group for the Advancement of Psychiatry (1995) goes a little further in calling for recognition in such classification systems of relational disorders which could be independent of individual pathology. Morbid jealousy may be among the conditions pertinent here and better considered as a relationship disorder (White and Mullen 1989), rather than necessarily a disorder in only one of the partners, even though one may have the principal pathology. While it is more likely than not that in a psychiatric hospital each individual does have relevant personal pathology, it is nevertheless important to consider that they may in addition have specific relationship problems that will require treatment. In a setting like a special hospital where domestic violence may have been a key factor in entry, this effort merely becomes more urgent.

COUPLES IN SPECIAL HOSPITAL: THE ISSUES FOR ASSESSMENT AND MANAGEMENT

Patient-Centred Issues

Among people with a psychotic illness, those with an affective psychosis are probably less disadvantaged than those with schizophrenia (the diagnosis of the majority in special hospitals) in their chances of finding a marital or marital type partner (Stevens 1969). Men with schizophrenia have been consistently shown to be less likely to form marital or stable marital-type relationships than women, probably because of the generally earlier onset of the disorder in men (Salokangas 1983; Test et al. 1990). There may be a special problem for the women too, however, in that they seem especially likely to have transitory relationships and chaotic sex lives (Miller and Finnerty 1996) and/or to attract violent men or men who have been diagnosed as having a personality disorder (Parnas 1985). Among the other risks may be the greater chance of personal violence. Several studies have now shown that within a sample of psychotic patients, those who engaged in personal violence were more likely to have a spouse than those who did not (Planansky and Johnston 1977; Häfner and Böker 1973), but then, given the isolation in the lives of many people with schizophrenia, this may be no more than an indicator of opportunity.

Then too, benefits as well as risks are clearly documented for marriage in which at least one partner has schizophrenia. In one substantial follow-up of patients who had left hospital, the only living arrangement to show a significant advantage for better health or staying out of hospital was marriage (Blumenthal et al. 1982). Nor is it necessarily the case that only those who have a better prognosis illness have an advantage in setting up home together. In a small British sample of people with chronic schizophrenia who had been counselled against marriage, but went ahead anyway, all showed significantly fewer symptoms and less disability in the two years after marriage than in the two years before (Shanks and Atkins 1985).

Personality disorder accounts for the disorders and disabilities of most of the other people resident in a special hospital and reference has already been made to the notion that relationship disorders are almost an intrinsic element. Particularly familiar in this setting is the 'incapacity to maintain enduring relationships, although no difficulties in establishing them' (ICD-10: dissocial personality disorder) and 'a liability to become involved in intense and unstable relationships' (ICD-10: borderline personality disorder).

Meriktangas (1982), reviewing the literature on 'assortative mating' – the tendency for individuals in a couple to be more similar for a particular characteristic than if the choice had occurred at random – concluded that it does occur for personality traits. The mechanism for this, however, remains unclear. Disorder may be limiting in the choice of partner as much by the environment in which it places the individual as by the disorder *per se*. Perhaps men with personality disorder and women with schizophrenia are particularly likely to pair because they are more likely to find themselves in the same social groups. Perhaps, too, repetition in relationships, for example of abusive qualities, is a reflection of prolonged experiences of abusing and dysfunctional relationships from childhood which were not only powerful but in their familiarity proved difficult to avoid or abandon in their entirety. Power imbalances established in childhood relationships may be perpetrated throughout adulthood; impairments in empathy and social perceptions, in some cases perhaps genetically influenced, in others perhaps learned, may persist.

Institutional Factors

Institutions by definition introduce rules and set limits. Residential institutions like prisons and hospitals limit choice of relationships by the regulations on who enters; they restrict the opportunities for relationships by the nature of accommodation, activities, staff monitoring and implicit and explicit rules. Any couple formation that may occur, however platonic, may raise anxieties and jealousies in a setting where people have disabilities in relationships and the needs of the community and safety of the individual are jointly paramount. The frequency of eroticised partnerships is unknown, but as lasting partnerships they are probably rare and, depending on the qualities of the individuals, may be regarded by staff and other residents as anywhere along the spectrum from normal to freakish. At any rate the intensity of the resulting observation, whether appropriate or not, may lend freakish qualities. Risks will be considered more fully elsewhere, but most are exaggerated by their institutional context. Violence holds an even greater horror because the managers of the institution have a responsibility to ensure safety; the ordinary risk of pregnancy if a relationship between a man and woman becomes sexual is exaggerated by the likelihood that effective contraception has been neither sought nor offered for a clandestine relationship.

The more regulated and more closed a community becomes, so choice of relationships becomes more limited. People who are already restricted by disabilities including severe social phobias or florid psychosis find that almost all their time is spent in the company of people with similar problems and they are cut off from the healthy. In an environment which includes offenders, then choices are further curtailed. The more secure or specialised the institution, the fewer places it provides and so the more likely it is that the individual will be geographically distanced from anyone that they have previously known. In some of the smaller medium secure hospital units it has been known that just one woman may occasionally have to co-exist on her own with 20–30 men; there are women on the staff, but she has no patient peer group. These institutional realities leave the individuals – men and women – with choices additionally generally restricted to same sex company.

It is rare in prisons for men and women to be held together, and even the possibility of mixing for some activities is unusual, affecting only a few centres in Europe. Where mixing occurs in the USA, evaluation suggests that it is appreciated by prisoners of both sexes (Cavior and Cohen 1980), although there remains a familiar concern that the needs of women, who are in a minority, are subordinated to those of the men (SchWeber 1984). Concern about abuse of women in prison has tended to focus on male officers rather than inmates (Human Rights Watch Women's Rights Project 1996).

In hospitals, including psychiatric hospitals, the same approach to segregation prevailed until the 'deinstitutionalisation' programmes in the mental hospitals of the 1950s. The concept of 'asylum' for people with chronic as well as acute disorders included rest from sexuality (Bourgeois 1975). Gender integration of living accommodation only reached two wards in the special hospital services, and one of those was for people with severe learning disabilities. While patients in other open psychiatric hospitals are beginning to call for and get segregated accommodation again, the principal point is that even in those secure institutions (hospitals or prisons) where some mixing is allowed, men outnumber women by four to one.

For those who do make contact with putative partners outside the institution there are even more unanswered questions – to do with the methods of approach and the qualities of people that respond. There are people who come forward unsolicited to befriend long-stay hospital patients or prisoners. There are people who have advertised themselves in magazines, often sexually explicit, who follow up a reply from patients or prisoners; there are those who respond to overt patient-initiated adverts. There is often some screening and even some supervision and support available to people who it is believed offer their time in a spirit of genuine altruism – but very little is known about their relative strengths, weaknesses or motives, of how they come to regard their task, of how much assistance they feel they need with it, how often they would rate their work or befriending as a success, or how often they may have felt threatened or had other problems. It is known that such relationships have developed romantically or erotically, but not how commonly so and almost nothing is known about how successful such developments may have been at least in terms of the mutual satisfaction of the couple, whether in the long or short term.

In this context some might argue that it is simply a good thing that opportunities for contact are limited – but the next question has to be: how are they limited? Again evidence is largely anecdotal, but the limits seem paradoxically to be directed maximally towards more healthy relationships. In prisons or secure hospitals, where relationships have survived the offence or dangerous act itself, the disincentives of geography, restricted visiting times, poor visiting accommodation, lack of specific facilities for children, strict observation of visits and so on are powerful disincentives. Clandestine relationships between prisoners or patients by definition are least restricted. This undoubtedly favours homosexuality regardless of the primary preference of the residents, and while it is important to be concerned about the exploitation of women by men, too little concern has been given to exploitation of women by women or men by men. Homosexual rape has been reported in psychiatric hospitals (Holbrook 1989) and in prisons (Nacci and Kane 1984).

In institutions where both men and women do co-exist staff are explicit that their greatest fear is of a pregnancy, and patients and staff alike observe that staff crack down on heterosexual partnerships but turn a blind eye to homosexual partnerships. On the rare occasion that prisoners or patients come forward to express their special seriousness about a relationship – to ask for special privileges or even marriage – a principal component of the staff response is to discourage and observe more closely.

THE FREQUENCY OF ROMANTIC OR SEXUAL RELATIONSHIPS IN SPECIAL HOSPITALS

No one knows how commonly people form close partnerships. At one extreme marriage is extremely rare. In cases where each of the partners is resident in a Special Hospital, marriages are in single figures at each. Where one partner is living outside, usually but not invariably in a marriage that has lasted from before admission, there are between ten and 30 at each hospital. There are other pairings, probably mainly among the people with personality disorder. Definitive figures are not available, but on one ward for 25 young men with personality disorder, a relationship of some importance and with practical management issues is the rule rather than the exception. Most favour relationships with young women with personality disorder also resident in the hospital, but one or two have relationships with women outside the hospital and one or two with other men inside the hospital. None is currently married.

The position for people with schizophrenia is more gloomy. In one series of 100 patients five had been living with a partner prior to the index offence that brought them into the special hospital, one of whom continued visiting. At the time of interview at varying periods into their admission nine of the men and seven of the women considered that they had a partner, four of the men claiming homosexual partnerships and all the others heterosexual. The majority of partners were also in a special hospital. At the other extreme, 25 per cent of this group of patients reported no social contacts at all, one third said they had no confidante and over 40 per cent no friends (Heads *et al.* in press).

Staff Factors

A non-systematic survey of staff and patient attitudes in special hospital revealed that staff were sometimes disapproving but mostly just afraid and feeling helpless in the face of an observed relationship. They thought they would be blamed for any untoward consequences of the relationship, had little or no concept of the possibility of benefit and felt so uncertain of their capacity to set limits that they preferred the 'blind eye' approach to a properly watchful brief. They were, however, willing to discuss the problems and asked some testing, practical questions. If we see two patients become exclusive in their relationship will the other patients react with jealousy or hostility? In one tragically unusual year there were two killings of one patient by another, both in the context of psychosis but also profound homosexual jealousy. If a patient confides details of a relationship that the clinical team of the other patient do not know about should we tell the other team or is that a breach of confidence? If we see two men kissing and fondling each other at a social, should we stop them?

A problem of which staff may be much less aware is the impact of their own relationships on patients. Patients commonly have unfounded fantasies about the nature and quality of relationships between staff but from time to time real staff relationships become the focus of interest. Transferences developing within therapeutic relationships may create jealousies, occasionally dangerous jealousy of the therapist's partner whether or not he or she works in the same organisation. New or clandestine relationships between staff members working on the same unit are seldom unrecognised by patients, and can give rise to pathological acting. In one instance, two members of staff who, in any direct sense behaved entirely properly to patients throughout, began an affair with each other. A flood of the male patients demanded the female staff member as their personal therapist, notwithstanding her lack of qualification for individual psychotherapeutic work. They considered her observed capacity for new relationship formation as an indication of her availability. A great deal of staff time was spent dealing with these requests, or complaints that the requests were not honoured.

One of the few absolutes in clinical (or pastoral) practice is that no person in a relationship of professional intimacy such as that between patient and doctor, therapist and patient, social worker and client, priest and confidante should eroticise that relationship or have sexual contact within it. The risks include harmful exploitation of the patient/client but also clouding of other aspects of professional judgement. Among clinicians this is partly to take account of the nature of physical contact sometimes necessary in order to practise effectively, and in mental health services it takes also special account of the nature of transferences that may develop, that is attachment of qualities that in many cases a patient is encouraged to transfer from other relationships to the therapeutic relationship. Such transference may be sexual, and the seductive power of some patients not to be underestimated. Therapists, however, are not invariably without problems themselves. Up to 8 per cent of psychiatrists alone, responding to anonymous surveys, have acknowledged sexual involvement with their patients (Garntrell et al. 1986). Psychiatrists who later treated such patients reported that the sexual contact was harmful to the patients (Garntrell et al. 1987). Only partly in jest Gonsiorek (1995) compares the US Food and Drug Administration (FDA) cut-off for banning a drug, at 1–2 per cent prevalence of serious adverse effects. If psychotherapy were a drug, he says, the FDA would be required to ban it simply on the basis of the high prevalence of this recognised adverse effect. Special Hospitals are no less vulnerable to such staff risks than any other therapeutic or closed community. In addition, as in many other hospitals, and much more extensively in prison, many people who are not professionally qualified assist in work with patients. They do not have professional codes, they have relatively little relevant training, and specific attention to practice guidelines and perhaps explicit contractual safeguards may be needed.

Training in the recognition of non-therapeutic behaviours with patients and the likelihood of their adverse effects is important, together with guidance on management. One useful practical indicator was offered by Feldbrugge (personal communication) from the Van der Hoerven Kliniek in Holland, for the treatment of people with personality disorder. If, as a member of staff, you notice elements in your relationship with a patient which you would rather another member of staff did not know about, you must seek supervision advice. At that clinic a staff member with a relationship recognised to have become eroticised will be offered the option between discontinuing the relationship with the patient and accepting professional counselling, or resigning. In the latter event s/he may then be treated as any other external friend of the patient. Even such an approach would not meet with universal approval. Appelbaum

and Jorgenson (1991) made an even more modest proposal that psychotherapist – patient sexual contact might be permitted one year after termination of
treatment, subject to the unequivocal wishes of both parties. It provoked the
largest correspondence the *American Journal of Psychiatry* had experienced at that
time, much of it deploring such a liberal view.

Outside Influences

One of the great difficulties in developing policy in sensitive areas in high profile institutions is that it can become 'news'. During the summer of 1994 one
tabloid newspaper used its entire front page to announce 'BROADMOOR
LOVE CHILD'. In what seemed a rare stroke of justice, soon after reporting this
fictional tale about a patient's pregnancy and the hospital's response, the newspaper ceased circulation.

More often, outside influences have been constructive. Specialist expertise
on many pertinent matters – the prevention and management of venereal infections, of HIV, of pregnancy, even given the extreme rarity of the former two and
no recorded evidence of the latter – is important in drawing up advance guidance. These are not tasks for which regular Special Hospital staff are qualified,
but they need to be prepared with basic training, and ready access to specialist
professional advice or supervision have been provided. Detained patients in
Special Hospital, as elsewhere, are perhaps uniquely placed among people in
regulated communities. They almost invariably have specialist advice of a different kind – their personal solicitor.

The risk of pregnancy, which had long preoccupied staff, was used to raise
awareness of child care issues more generally. This should necessarily involve
external agencies on behalf of the children. It is not certainly known how many
special hospital patients have children; it is recognised from attempts to establish need among prisoners and their families that women in such situations are
particularly likely to be the sole caretakers of their children, and have a tendency to conceal information about their children through fear of official interference in their child care arrangements. Just over 20 per cent of the men and
nearly one third of the women under 50 and living in special hospital declared
children to the research register (Ferraro *et al.* in press). Notwithstanding the
confidentiality of this data collection we suspect this is an underestimate. Nevertheless, if all operated well, local authorities nationwide would be in contact
with the hospitals about the care of dependent children of at least 250 male and
63 female patients.

The other main practical input, particularly important for those many patients who have no family or community support, is from non-statutory bodies
and pressure groups, such as Women in Special Hospital (WISH), a sister organisation of Women in Prison (WIP), and the Matthew Trust. They variously

offer direct advice to management, solicited and unsolicited, visit and support the patients, encourage patients to advocate and act for themselves in the hospitals and generally seek to raise awareness about rights.

MANAGING RELATIONSHIPS: THE TASKS

Recognition

Accurate observation is the most important skill in the successful management of relationships – as of almost anything else. This includes formally noting exactly what people say and do in any given situation, the circumstance of that situation and what is already known about those people; only then can an effective judgement be made about the nature and quality of any relationship and any necessary management planning begin.

Many factors work against this idea in institutional settings. Because anxiety about relationships developing the potential for sexual expression is so general, staff may be as enthusiastic as patients that such relationships remain covert. Staff feel unprepared in their training or numbers for the complexity of judgements and intervention they may have to make over time, and confident only in a complete bar on any physicality that becomes inescapably overt. Management structures tend principally to be critical of failures of affirmative action and to accept more readily that preliminaries were not seen or consummation not foreseen, and so inadvertently reinforce this denial.

There is also a risk of mistaken emphasis in what need and need not be recognised. Staff may correctly judge that a relationship is likely to be transitory, but this does not thereby carry an implication that it can safely be ignored. In institutions, as elsewhere, some risks, including unprotected sexual intercourse, are at their highest in transient relationships. Among those who are vulnerable to exploitation, people are as likely to be damaged by an immediate intrusion as one that is planned and delayed. Each of the phases of a relationship – its making, maintenance and end – is likely to need attention. Transient relationships simply have fewer of the maintenance needs.

Assessment

At the heart of assessment is continued but now more focused observation as the means to complete a risk–benefit analysis of an identified relationship, which will, in turn, inform effective management. Table 12.1 sets out some of the principal areas that staff and patients alike see as important elements in such an assessment. For almost each area there is a spectrum from risk to benefit, and, as relationships change over time, it is important that each is regularly monitored. A relationship which one day may have been beneficial in making a pa-

Table 12.1 Patient relationships in a special hospital: some perceived risks and benefits

	Risks	Benefits
Physical Health	Pregnancy Infection	Increased self-esteem Increases self-care and health promotion interests
	Assault Sexual exploitation Self-harm	Mutual support in disengagement from harmful practice
	Habit sharing e.g. drug use	
Mental Health	*Direct*	
	Increased stress Relapse of disorder Emergence of PTSD-type reactions	Decreased isolation and stress Increased well-being/self-esteem
	Indirect	
	Less individuality Denial of personal problems 'Flight into normality'	Increased treatment compliance New courses for treatment e.g. couples therapy Opportunities to practise new skills
Social	Hostility of un-paired peers Jealousy of the previously paired Damage to other fragile relations e.g. family Prurient staff/media interest	Respect after previous isolation More in common with outside family/friends Successful relationships increase longer-term stability

tient feel attractive and wanted may, even after some disagreement that appears trivial to staff, leave that individual feeling rejected, despairing and suicidal.

Sometimes it is not immediately apparent where the element fits on the risk–benefit spectrum. As indicated, many of the patients – men and women – have suffered extensive abuse in previous intimate relationships, and have expressed their anger in various forms of self and other abuse. A new intimate relationship in an environment such as a Special Hospital thus carries both the risk of further actual abuse and the resurgence of powerful negative emotions, as any intimacy may be coloured with abusive or supposed abusive qualities. Superficially both these effects are simple risks from which the patient needs protection. The latter, however, can prove to be a benefit, enabling the patient for the first time to disclose earlier abuse and begin the process of working through its consequences. There was an early lesson in this process for staff on the unit at Ashworth Hospital where 12 men and 12 women share residential accommodation. The staff had prepared themselves to recognise and intervene in any physical approaches between the men and women. True the patients had been assessed prior to their transfer there as unlikely to make such approaches, but in any event the staff had little call on their prepared skills. What was unexpected and required new direction in skill acquisition, was the flow of people coming forward for the first time to disclose earlier abuse.

In so far as patients exploit their romantic and erotic relationships, that too is generally at rather more subtle levels than commonly expected. Some patients, for example, have used relationships, whether consciously or not, as a means of shifting responsibility for their own continuing anti-social behaviour or unhappiness or as a means of denying personal problems. Individual therapy or treatment programmes are rejected in favour only of activities that will ensure meetings with the beloved. Occasionally a new relationship is itself used as a hostile act to another patient who may have previously 'dated' the new partner, and then it can be vital to understand the full extent of social networks of each person involved – within and outside the hospital – to ensure safety. A major concern in any institution where for some a preferred method of solving relationship problems is violence, is invariably physical safety. Self-harm in this context is as likely to be an act of violence to the partner or others as to be pure self-destructiveness.

Management

A large hospital setting has many advantages over smaller hospital units, hostels or prisons for the management of relationships. It provides greater opportunity for wide-ranging input and the provision of appropriate proximity or distance. Greater opportunities, however, can be foiled by poor communication. Clarity and documentation of the management plan together with guidance on monitoring its effects are an essential preliminary to dissemination. Set dates for review as well as *ad hoc* arrangements will be necessary. Although many staff may need information about the situation, it may not be appropriate for, say, a technical assistant in an occupational therapy area to have the same amount as one patient's primary nurse, or for one patient's clinical team to have as much information personal to the other's clinical team as that other team. A dilemma arises if the patients share a psychiatrist or clinical team. It is probably best, if a relationship appears to have long-term potential, that each patient has an independent set of clinicians, such that each can be confident that the team will act in his or her best interests, regardless of the outcome of the relationship.

For a few relationships the risk–benefit analysis will tip so far towards risk that management will require separation, or at the least continuous conspicuous supervision while the couple are together. Few relationship contracts in such settings are likely to last indefinitely. There is no information on informal relationships, but my impression is that few endure more than a few months. Of eight Special Hospital marriages contracted between 1983 and 1990, three had failed by 1991. Managing the separation is as important as managing a surviving relationship, whatever the reason for its discontinuance. This will mean support for each person as an individual, but may also include joint work. If that can be achieved, for some of the patients in Special Hospital this may be a particularly valuable experience as the first time they have felt/been able to assert themselves in ending a relationship without violence.

Availability of General Guidance

While each relationship must be treated as unique and the assessment and management plan tailored for the special circumstances, both patients/residents and staff benefit from guidance on the context in which that can and will be done. While recognising anachronisms in the expectation of sexual continence in a long-term residential population, more than 80 per cent of whom are under 50, sexual continence nevertheless is the expectation of all hospitals and prisons in Britain. Written policies seem exceptionally hard to agree in this field, but taken in the spirit that they will need regular formal review, are essential. Detailed practice guidelines are much more a matter for each case. While the expectation has to be clear, and while it must thus be enforced as far as possible, staff have to balance this with realism. It is extremely unlikely that all sexual activity can be prevented even in a highly supervised secure institution, so responsibilities arise for other sorts of prevention – against pregnancy and transmission of contact infections. Policy must take account of anachronisms between, for example, 'we don't allow it, but we are giving you the means of protection because we think it could happen' and 'homosexual acts in a public place are forbidden by law, secure hospitals/prisons are public places, to provide condoms there is to be an accessory in breaking the law; but to fail to provide reasonable protection against a real risk is to be liable for harm befalling a resident'.

Even the unlikeliest of possible events must be allowed for if safety is to be maximised. A patient pregnancy, for example, has not yet occurred in the special hospitals, but it is not impossible. If this should be suspected, immediate action to safeguard the interests of the possible child, and then each parent, is essential. Under the Children Act 1989 every child's interests are paramount and agencies with specific responsibility for such a child would be involved individually on confirmation of a pregnancy.

Staff Support and Supervision

The existence of general guidance is in itself a form of support for staff, but other forms of support and supervision are necessary too if they are to be effective in any sensitive and hitherto largely uncharted areas. Some of the support will naturally emerge from the teamwork which is common practice, but some of the supervision will ideally be drawn from experienced experts. As indicated earlier, this is easier said than achieved, but in prolonged work with couples at the least a more distant professional input to monitoring its effect is likely to be helpful.

Apart from agreement on the general principles of a management plan for a couple – whether the relationship is to be facilitated, merely tolerated and observed or ended – some detailing of the practical arrangements will be important. In secure institutions of any kind the limits to privacy, for example, must be specified – to what extent may letters or phone calls be unmonitored and how closely supervised should visits be? What special arrangements if any must be adopted? It is important that decisions on contraception and sexual health are taken openly, and not by default, and any specific counselling or treatment needs will need to be identified.

OTHER MODELS

Worldwide, limits are set on the extent to which personal relationships may be fulfilled within institutional settings. A sense of concern about risks between potential sexual partners in secure institutions, and perhaps particularly in secure hospitals, is truly international. The sanctions against heterosexual relationships tend to be more explicit than those against homosexual relationships in a reversal of common anxieties brought about by a general prejudice in the law in favour of heterosexuality. Nevertheless, not all countries practice the same limits. While in Britain there is no sanctioned conjugal visiting within prison or hospitals, and even hostels or community homes seem resistant to it, a few countries have such settings which do offer carefully monitored possibilities. Most, like Britain, notionally have policies which allow infrequently for certain prisoners, usually towards the end of a sentence, to have weekend leave for conjugal purposes if the relationship has managed to survive to that point. For detained patients similarly, if more rarely relevant, this becomes possible if very stable and out of high security. In Denmark, however, both a psychiatric prison (Hevsdedvester) and a high security hospital (Nykøping) allow residents who are stable to meet in complete privacy in the prison/hospital with their spouses if they have them. In Holland, too, in therapeutic units, particularly those for the treatment of personality disorder, staff view conjugal visits within the secure perimeter as an important part of the rehabilitation package at an appropriate stage in the treatment.

CONCLUSIONS

Psychiatry has a long history of muddled thinking about associations between intimate or sexual relationships and mental disorder, with or without accompanying dangerous acts. Nevertheless, there is good reason to consider both the impact of relationships on disorder and the safety of relationships in the context of it. In secure settings, here secure hospitals, special attention is needed because of the special responsibility of the hospitals for the safety of the patients, and staff and public, and because of the disproportionate risks of harm in close relationships where at least one of the partners is a patient who has already been violent. This should not, however, obscure the possibility that even here such relationships can be highly beneficial. If benefit is to outweigh risks, general policies and guidance on management and individualised planning are needed. With little real knowledge and only slightly more experience, such guidance is necessarily in its infancy, but has been offered here if only to further discussion.

REFERENCES

Appelbaum, P.S. and Jorgenson, L.M. (1991) 'Psychotherapist–patient sexual contact after termination of treatment.' *American Journal of Psychiatry 148*, 1466–1473.

Blumenthal, R., Kreisman, D. and O'Connor, P. (1982) 'Return to the family and its consequence for rehospitalisation among recently discharged mental patients.' *Psychological Medicine 12*, 141–147.

Bourgeois, M. (1975) 'Sexualité et Institution Psychiatrique.' *Evolution Psychiatrique 40*, 551–573.

Cavior, H.E. and Cohen, S.H. (1980) 'The development of a scale to assess inmate and staff attitudes toward co-corrections.' In J.O. Smykla (ed) *Coed Prison*. New York: Human Sciences Press

Committee on the Family, Group for the Advancement of Psychiatry (1995) 'A model for the classification and diagnosis of relational disorder.' *Psychiatric Services 46*, 926–931.

Duggan, C. 'Couples' assessment' (in press) In P.J. Taylor and T. Swann (eds) *Couples in Care and Custody*. Butterworth Heinemann: Oxford.

Feldbrugge, J.T.T.M. (Personal communication) Van der Hoerven Kliniek, Postbus 174, Willem Dresslaan 2, Utrecht, Netherlands.

Ferraro, D., Kennedy, M., Leese, M. and Taylor, P.J. (submitted) 'Are national principles and the care programme approach likely to be enough?' (Available from the authors at the Institute of Psychiatry, London SE5 8AF).

Fitzgerald, E. and Harbour, A. (in press) 'Marriages and partnerships for psychiatric patients or prisoners: European rights and the law in England and Wales.' In P.J. Taylor and T. Swann (eds) *Couples in Care and Custody*. Butterworth Heinemann: Oxford.

Gartrell, N., Herman, J., Olarte, S., Feldstein, M. and Localio, R. (1986) 'Psychiatrist–patient sexual contact: results of a national survey. I: prevalence.' *American Journal of Psychiatry 143*: 1126–1131.

Gartrell, N., Herman, J., Olarte, S., Feldstein, M. and Localio, R. (1987) 'Reporting practice of psychiatrists who knew of sexual misconduct by colleagues.' *American Journal of Psychiatry 57*, 287–296.

Gonsiorek, J.C. (ed) (1995) *Breach of Trust. Sexual Exploitation by Health Care Professionals and Clergy*. Thousand Oaks, CA: Sage.

Gordon, H. (in press) 'International perspectives on the theory and practice of sexuality in secure institutions.' In P.J. Taylor and T. Swann (eds) *Couples in Care and Custody*. Butterworth Heinemann: Oxford.

Häfner, H. and Böker, W. (1973), (translated by H. Marshall, 1982) *Crimes of Violence by Mentally Abnormal Offenders*. Cambridge: Cambridge University Press.

Heads, T., Leese, M., Taylor, P.J. and Phillips, S. (submitted) 'A special hospital sample of patients with schizophrenia: social integration, aspects of illness and violent behaviour.' (Available from the authors at the Institute of Psychiatry, London SE5 8AF).

Holbrook, T. (1989) 'Policing sexuality in a modern state hospital.' *Hospital and Community Psychiatry 40*, 75–79.

Human Rights Watch Women's Rights Project (1996) *All Too Familiar: Sexual Abuse of Women in U.S. State Prisons*. New York: Human Rights Watch.

Laumann, E.O., Gagnon, J.H., Michael, R.T. and Michaels, S. (1994) *The Social Organization of Sexuality: Sexual Practices in the United States*. Chicago: University of Chicago Press.

Lewontin, R.C. (1995) 'Sex, lies and social science.' *The New York Review of Books XLII*, 24–29.

Merikangas, K.R. (1982) 'Assortative mating for psychiatric disorders and psychological traits.' *Archives of General Psychiatry 39*, 173–1180.

Miller, L.J. and Finnerty, M. (1996) 'Sexuality, pregnancy, and child rearing among women with schizophrenia-spectrum disorders.' *Psychiatric Services 47*, 502–506.

Mulligan, T. and Moss, C.R. (1991) 'Sexuality and aging in male veterans: a cross-sectional study of interest, ability and activity.' *Archives of Sexual Behavior 20*, 17–25.

Nacci, P.L. and Kane, T.R. (1984) 'Sex and sexual aggression in federal prisons: inmate involvement and employee impact.' *Federal Probation 40*, 46–53.

Parnas, J. (1985) 'Mates of schizophrenic mothers; a study of assortative mating from the American–Danish High Risk Project.' *British Journal of Psychiatry 146*, 490–497.

Pfeiffer, E., Verwerdt, A. and Wang, H.S. (1969) 'The natural history of sexual behaviour in a biologically advantaged group of aged individuals.' *Journal of Gerontology 24*, 193–198.

Planansky, K. and Johnston, R. (1977) 'Homicidal aggression in schizophrenic men.' *Acta Psychiatrica Scandinavica 55*, 65–73.

Salokangas, R.K.R. (1983) 'Prognostic implications of the sex of schizophrenic patients.' *British Journal of Psychiatry 142*, 145–151.

Schweber, C. (1984) 'Beauty marks and blemishes: the coed prison as a microcosm of integrated society.' *Prison Journal 64*, 3–14.

Shanks, J. and Atkins, P. (1985) 'Psychiatric patients who marry each other.' *Psychological Medicine 15*, 377–382.

Skynner, R. (1980) 'Recent developments in marital therapy.' *The Journal of Family Therapy 2*, 271–296.

Stevens, B.C. (1969) *Marriage and Fertility of Women Suffering from Schizophrenia or Affective Disorders*. Maudsley Monograph, No. 19. London: Oxford University Press.

Taylor, P.J., Leese, M., Williams, D., Butwell, M., Daly, R., Larkin, E. and others in the Special Hospitals' Treatment Resistant Schizophrenia Group (1998). 'Mental Disorder and Violence: A Special Hospital Study.' *British Journal of Psychiatry 172*, 218–226.

Test, M.A., Burke, S.S. and Wallischls (1990) 'Gender differences of young adults with schizophrenic disorders in community care.' *Schizophrenia Bulletin 16*, 331–344.

Wharton, E. (1920) *The Age of Innocence Now*. Dent: London.

White, G.L. and Mullen, P.E. (1989) *Jealousy, Theory, Research and Clinical Strategies*. New York: Guildford Press.

WHO (1992) *The ICD-10 Classification of Mental and Behavioural Disorders*. World Health Organisation: Geneva.

CASES CITED

Draper v United Kingdom D and R [1981] (Page 95). United Kingdom.

Hamer v United Kingdom D and R [1981] (Page 95). United Kingdom.

Park, In the Estate of [1953] 2 All ER 1411; [1v. Park [1054] Page 112 at 127.

X and Y v. Switzerland Application No. 8166/78 D and R [1979] Page 242.

PART 4

Accelerating Change

CHAPTER 13

Special Hospitals and Change

A Chaplain Reflects

Trevor Walt

INTRODUCTION

This chapter may appear a little different from the rest. In part, like other contributors, I simply intend to describe what has happened to one Special Hospital in recent years, but in addition I hope to offer some kind of personal, spiritual reflection on the whole nature of the Special Hospital and on the effects of change upon it over a longer time scale.

Special Hospitals are very special places. They are reflections of the rest of society, representing the darkest possibilities of the human condition and at the same time, the highest ideals of humanity. Their very existence both confirms our greatest fears of what human beings are capable of and yet reassures us that we live in an ordered society where the disordered are treated well and somewhat differently to those who are just considered bad. The hospitals are, however, and have always been, something of a paradox. When attempting to trace the origins of this, we return to the year 1800. In that year a man called James Hadfield attempted to kill King George III whilst he attended the Dury Lane Theatre. Hadfield had been discharged from the Army because of insanity, caused by a head wound. At his trial he used the classic delusional defence to explain his behaviour. He claimed that God had commanded him to do it! It was, of course, fortuitous that Hadfield was known by the Royal Family (he had been Orderly to the Duke of York) and that he was so obviously insane, for otherwise he might well have gone to the gallows. Instead, the Judge, Lord Kenyon, instructed the jury to find him 'not guilty by reason of insanity' and even more importantly, stated that he should be 'cared for, all mercy and humanity being shown'.

This one event describes the origin of the paradox well. Hadfield was found 'not guilty' by reason of insanity, but he had committed the act! The Judge ordered that he should be 'cared for' but how and where? Several days later, Parliament swiftly passed the Insanity Bill of 1800, making provision for the verdict and for persons so found to be kept in strict custody until 'His Majesty's pleasure be known' and Hadfield went back to Newgate Prison because there was nowhere else. From then until now there has been a constant political, legal and medical debate about the care, custody and treatment of persons like Hadfield. It took half a century of such debate before the existence of the paradox was accepted and recognised well enough to enable the creation of an asylum especially designed for the purpose.

1863 AND BEYOND: A PARADOX BECOMES REALITY

In 1863, Broadmoor Criminal Lunatic Asylum was opened in Berkshire, controlled and managed by the Home Office, but even then seen to be distinctly unique and not part of the Prison Service. It was founded upon the strong Christian ethic prevalent in the middle Victorian era and its Chapel and Chaplain were given due prominence from the beginning. It was set apart from the rest of society but represented imaginative and forward thinking in its design and operation. Men and women detained under the earlier legislation in prisons and madhouses throughout the whole of the country were moved to Broadmoor in 1863 and 1864 and by all accounts, they were 'cared for, all mercy and humanity being shown'. The paradox was now a visible reality.

Over 100 years later, I found myself entering the gates of Broadmoor Hospital in 1971. I had been attracted by an advertisement in the national press for student psychiatric nurses in the Special Hospital Service. All of the Special Hospitals were approved centres for full Registered Nurse Training at that time and I remember well the glossy brochure which I received with the application form. It described, in 1971, the rapidly developing therapeutic environment of a modern psychiatric institution wrestling with, inevitably, the balance between security and treatment. There was an expanding nurse education programme designed to equip professional nurses to care for the patient population within. Having given up a place in higher education, I arrived at Broadmoor which was even then considered to be a specialist centre with a long historical tradition of the care and management of the mentally abnormal offender and with an infamous national and international reputation. I was 19 years old and very inexperienced but soon realised that I had, in fact, enrolled at what could only be described as a 'red brick' university of life.

On reflection and with the wonderful vision of hindsight, it is obvious to me that at the time I arrived, Broadmoor was very much an institution still trapped by the vagaries and traditions of history. It had no doubt changed since its creation in 1863 but only by a process of slow evolution, nothing radical ever occurring. The lines of the Authority within the Hospital at that time were very clear. Power lay primarily in the hands of the Physician Superintendent, who was ably supported by the Head of Nursing and an Administrator. Up until that time, most staff recruitment had been from the local population and often from within existing families, many of whom had proudly worked for the institution for several generations.

The hospital provided nurse training, guarantee of future employment after qualification, housing for married staff, extra pay in the form of a Special Hospital lead payment and a level of job security and pension rights, which amounted to nothing less than the principle of a 'job for life'. In return, staff were mostly content with their conditions of service, felt very secure and, above all, tended to offer what amounted to total loyalty to the hospital. The relationship between employer and employee was paternalistic and increasingly unrealistic in the second half of the twentieth century, but was based on a model of operation which had been successful for over 100 years.

With major changes beginning to occur in the wider NHS, it was obvious that Broadmoor could not continue as a backwater of Victorian paternalism. Some things had already changed; the second half of the century had begun with a Royal Commission resulting in the Mental Health Act of 1959; conventional hospitals had thrown open their doors; new treatments were proving to have amazing effect in unlocking the complex needs of chronically ill patients and as a consequence, only Broadmoor and the other Special Hospitals were destined to remain major places of detention for the mentally ill. As a result of legal changes, Broadmoor became vastly overcrowded in the 1970s, attempting to care for over 800 patients in space our Victorian predecessors felt was suitable for no more than 500. This did little else than concentrate the negative aspects of institutional life. Broadmoor survived many difficult times during these years, but remained nonetheless a relatively calm and well-ordered place. The balance between security and treatment was continually questioned as newer treatment approaches were developed, but the principle seemed to remain unchanged. Unlike similar institutions in other countries with separate security and treatment staff, the British Special Hospitals have always operated with one genre of staff with the dual responsibility of custody and caring. The overriding principle that I was taught, both in my formal nurse training and by experience, was that, once agreed, the level of physical security in the hospital was accepted by all as unchangeable. It was often quite surprising how much flexibility could be afforded to any treatment approach attempted within.

In the late 1970s and early 1980s, the patient overcrowding was relieved by the building of Park Lane (now Ashworth) Hospital and by the gradual development of Regional Secure Facilities. Broadmoor then steadily headed towards the newer and bigger challenge of developing services to come into line with the reforms of the wider NHS.

It is now clear that, accepting that challenge, steady evolution, however comfortable it may be for staff, would never have brought about the levels of change required nor the corresponding change in culture necessary of the staff in order for Broadmoor to become a first-class provider of high security psychiatric services. Radical change was necessary and the details and extent of the changes are fully documented elsewhere in this book. My interest continues to be the effects of change on the whole hospital community and upon individuals within it.

1988 AND BEYOND: THE EFFECTS OF CHANGE

I became fully responsible for the provision of Chaplaincy needs at Broadmoor Hospital in October 1988. I had already been employed by the hospital for 17 years as a nurse and nurse tutor and consequently was, myself, a product of the paternalism which had reigned for so long. I was now to be a Pastor, both to patients I had nursed and to colleagues I had taught and worked with. Initially I was very concerned about the prospect of being beleaguered by conflicts arising from my change of status, but very soon realised this was not to be. On the contrary, I felt totally supported by the whole community and settled quickly to a ministry that, although complex and all-absorbing, has proved to be very rewarding.

At that time, the hospital continued to function on one level as it always had, surviving slings and arrows, but on another level, there was an increasing unease and a growing powerful feeling that an era was coming to an end. Other commentators have described well the hospital's inadequacies, both clinically and organisationally, during the last years of the 1980s. In response to these, radical changes to the hospital environment and reform of the role and function of clinical teams were initiated.

In relation to the hospital environment, the commissioning of new buildings including wards, medical centre, physical care unit and a dedicated male admission ward was the greatest change since the original building of the institution. This was the first phase of what was to have been a major rebuilding programme which could not continue because of capital funding restrictions. Attention was drawn instead to the upgrading of existing buildings and for many patients and staff, this programme of redevelopment with the resulting ending of 'slopping out' has been of even greater value to the hospital.

A further change in hospital practice which has had a profound effect on patient care and behaviour has been the programme of male/female integration. Daytime therapeutic and social activities in the hospital are now patient integrated and all wards and departments are now male/female staff integrated. Although there have been some concerns about risk assessment and safety in relation to integration, the overall benefits in terms of patient behaviour and therapeutic care are significant.

All these changes have had positive effect on the work of the Chaplaincy. When I became Chaplain, it was very unlikely that a clinical team would invite me to discuss the individual needs of a patient. Today, I am considered to be an honorary member of every clinical team and have open access to patient care planning where necessary. For several years there has been a growing willingness among staff to assist in the assessing and meeting of patient spiritual and worship needs.

One of the symbols of institutional life which I inherited was the rule that patients could only sit in chapel in rows designated by ward. This practice was archaic, counter-therapeutic and not conducive to patterns of worship. Although some staff were anxious, it was decided on one particular Sunday in 1989 to allow patients, both male and female, to sit wherever they liked and no major difficulties have been experienced.

Overall, the benefits of change to the environment and to patient care can be summed up by quoting the answer to a question I put recently to a patient who was re-admitted to the hospital after a gap of 16 years. I asked him if he could tell me what had changed and he said 'Broadmoor seems now to have the ambience of a hospital and not a place of custody'. This one comment is truly symbolic of the gains that have been made.

The effects of change upon hospital staff have in some ways been more complex. In 1988, as Chaplain, my general perception of staff was of an increased level of uncertainty and fearfulness. For the first time in the hospital's long history, the practice of promoting the most senior staff from within, especially in the nursing discipline, had come to an end. For the first time generic managers were brought into the organisation at the highest levels and it took time for staff fully to appreciate the meaning of this.

During a very short time-scale the former management arrangements of the Hospital were replaced with a 'task-force', clearly signifying both a break from the past and a perception of the magnitude of the job in hand to begin Broadmoor's transformation. For several years the rest of the NHS had been moving rapidly down the path of reform so that the perceived gap between a new-style NHS Trust Hospital and a Special Hospital had widened even further than it had always been. The task of our new managers, and later the SHSA, was to set about reforming the organisation and clinical practice of Broadmoor Hospital to narrow this gap and encourage a major shift in the attitudes and culture of staff.

Not surprisingly, there have been casualties among staff along the way. Many staff, particularly those approaching the twilight years of their service, have felt a little adrift in a sea of change and have sought retirement earlier than they might have done. Some younger staff have become frustrated and disillu-

sioned by change leading to resistance and poor levels of job satisfaction. However, a larger number of staff, whether or not they have always agreed with
changes proposed, have displayed professional resilience leading them to new
and fruitful opportunities within the organisation.

The nature of reform and, moreover, the rapid rate of change have led some
staff to criticise managers in ways with which I can truly empathise. In the
whole of the NHS, and equally in all public service, there has been a major shift
towards devolution of managerial and budgetary authority to the lowest levels
of an organisation together with a corresponding increase in individual, professional accountability for all staff. In parallel, British society has moved considerably towards an ethic of individual rights as seen in the advent of patient and
other consumer charters. The result of this at the 'coal-face' of the Special Hospital has been that the risk of conflict between the rights of individual patients
and the responsibilities and duty of care of the staff has become more acute.
This has sometimes led to staff feeling professionally impotent with a corresponding lowering of morale.

Considering the nature of our patient population it is not surprising that
critical incidents occur. Two examples of incidents which have the most serious
effect on the hospital community are an escape and a suicide. When a patient
escapes, the response of all staff is immediate and the hospital's record for both
preventing and resolving such incidents is good. Every escape requires careful
investigation into what occurred and whether or not policies, practices or the
action of individuals were at fault. Individual staff who may have been involved
in any breakdown of security inevitably feel a great weight of responsibility
and in my experience are always riddled with feelings of guilt even when they
know that their actions were not directly culpable. At such times, staff need a
very high level of care and support, especially if they find themselves temporarily suspended from duty. Managers and all staff must do whatever they can to
dispel the notion of a 'blame culture' and this is best achieved by the whole organisation accepting overall responsibility corporately. We should all feel
equally responsible for both the hospital's success and failures.

Incidents resulting in suicide are in some way similar but involve staff not
just suffering from feelings of responsibility, but also wrestling with the process
of grief, both for their patients and themselves. Since my appointment as Chaplain, I have ministered to patients, their families and staff at the scene and aftermath of nine suicides and in the midst of what is always a tragedy, I can report
that a growing awareness has developed whereby patients and staff alike are
more able to express their grief and seek support when required. This process, I
believe, has been greatly enhanced by whole ward communities being willing
to attend funerals and memorial services in the Hospital Chapel.

Overall, whilst supporting the drive towards individual, professional accountability among staff, I would urge managers to assist staff in not losing

sight of the great benefits of facing all the changes and challenges of hospital life corporately with the mutual support of one another.

As for the speed of change, there has been an exponential effect. Sometimes the rate of change in our hospital over recent years has led me to pray for things to slow down a little; for one reorganised structure to last a little longer before the next one is proposed; for deadlines to be a little longer and for goals to be a little more achievable. It never ceases to amuse me that, in a hospital where the average length of stay and programme of care for a patient can be as long as 7–10 years, we can only plan a contract with our new purchasers for one year! We seem to accept too readily that the short-termism operating in a general hospital with an average length of stay of two days is easily transferable to the environment of a Special Hospital.

1997–2000 AND BEYOND: WHAT NEXT?

The reforms of recent years have brought many benefits to the life of Broadmoor Hospital and yet there has been a price to pay as described. The long-term future of the Special Hospitals is not entirely clear as we approach the end of the century and it is natural to wonder what further changes may occur. There has always been a natural tendency for each generation of carers and managers to strive to do better than the last and although we may be proud of what we have achieved, future generations of staff at Broadmoor Hospital will, no doubt, find good reasons to criticise us. The operational practices which we believe to be at the cutting edge of forensic mental health care today may well be bluntly looked upon with scorn by the professional eyes of tomorrow. The jargon of today will be quickly overtaken by the jargon of tomorrow and this is the nature of professional life. We can be relatively sure, however, that the care needs of the patients of the future will be remarkably similar to those of today, just as the needs of James Hadfield in 1800 were similar to patients that I cared for in the 1970s. Some things remain unchanged and relatively unchangeable. In my ministry today, in the ministry of predecessors and in the ministry of any Christian Chaplain of the future, meeting the basic spiritual needs of patients and staff has remained and will remain unchanged. Above all, for me, the forever unchanging element will always be the permanent and loving presence of Almighty God. We may now belong to a health care market in which everything is costed but God is the eternal accountant, our ultimate purchaser and provider. He purchased for us, by the sacrifice of his Son, the way of salvation for us all whether patient or staff and he provides for us all we will ever need to feel valued and fulfil our purpose in life. At this present moment in the history of our hospital, the responsibility for exercising stewardship over this part of creation falls to us, the current generation of staff. As long as we believe in what we do and can justify our actions, we can rest assured that history will at least judge us with respect.

It would, however, be wise for us occasionally to stand back, reflect, and take what I simply like to refer to as the 'longer' view of life. When I do this, I cannot help feeling that after such a major period of change in the life of the hospital it may now be right to rest awhile and take stock of where we are and where we have come from. If we do not, it is just possible that we may be in danger of attempting to achieve too much too quickly and then achieve nothing at all. The ability of human beings to reflect intellectually this way is less to do with knowledge and more to do with wisdom and if we are seeking to act wisely, I make no apology for quoting from my favourite book of the Old Testament, the Book of Ecclesiastes, which is part of what is commonly referred to as Wisdom Literature in the Bible.

> There is a time for everything and a season for every activity under heaven:
>
> a time to be born and a time to die
>
> a time to plant and a time to uproot
>
> a time to kill and a time to heal
>
> a time to tear down and a time to build.
>
> (Ecclesiastes, Chapter 3, Verses 1–8)

The first half of the nineteenth century was a time for some of the most able physicians, lawyers and social reformers to recognise the needs of a special group of disordered people and begin providing for their care with 'all mercy and humanity being shown'. For more than 100 years there was a time for Broadmoor to remain relatively static; a time for institutional care and custody which led, sadly, to some institutional stagnation. Recent years have undoubtedly been a time for rapid reform to help Broadmoor Hospital to become a major forensic mental health provider in a modern National Health Service.

As we rapidly approach a new millennium, could it be that now may be a time to rest and consolidate the gains we have made in both the philosophy and practices of our care giving; a time not to be perpetually looking for something new, but just to allow what is new to grow?

I began by stating that I hoped to offer a personal, spiritual reflection and I apologise for going further and making the assumption that as Chaplain I am allowed to be prophetic in some way, but as the writer of Ecclesiastes also states: 'There is a time to be silent and a time to speak'.

CHAPTER 14

Freedom from Restraint

Frank Powell

THE BACKGROUND

Both the wide literature regarding mental institutions, and the many enquiry reports and reviews specific to the special hospitals, describe patterns of staff behaviour and presentation which have been characterised as punitive or custodial and only occasionally therapeutic. A continuum of practice may be described ranging from incarceration to that which can be identified as liberal and enlightened. The six objectives established for the SHSA in 1989 epitomise the latter end of this continuum. Although, in 1989, emphases varied, there was ample evidence of punitive, custodial and therapeutic approaches to care and treatment.

PUNITIVE ATTITUDES

Punitive, or coercive, approaches are indicated by direct control measures, for example, locking up or physical restraint, or indirect measures such as the use of threat or sanctions. Whilst special hospitals are essentially required to be externally highly secure there was much evidence that internal regimes were also more closely based upon a 'prison' rather than 'hospital' model. Patients were locked in their room or dormitory at night from 9pm to 7am. Methods of physical control were regularly applied in the form of seclusion, the use of restraint garments and excessive medication. Staff who maintained punitive attitudes were liable to use such forms of physical control in combination with verbal threats and the abusive use of 'privilege systems'. They either had no concept of the patient as an individual with human needs and emotions or felt that the patient was not deserving of such consideration. Therefore there was no meaningful care planning, no interest in therapy or the benefits the patient might obtain through participation, and no concept of or interest in rehabilitative processes. There was little regard for the ward environment, which remained austere and formal, and scant consideration for the patient's need for privacy and self-respect. Practices and timetables were highly regimented. The ward culture was the domain of nursing staff and this was keenly protected from 'external influences' whether they be clinical staff with a responsibility for patients on the ward, managers or other visitors.

The punitive model had been organisationally reinforced for many years through the designation and abuse of 'refractory', 'special care' or 'intensive care' units. These areas were used for patients to be admitted, or transferred to, when demonstrating a high degree of dangerousness, or perceived potential dangerousness, to themselves or others. The operational need for such units was not clearly established as the proportion of such designated beds varied significantly between hospitals. The written objective for one unit included '...to attempt to achieve sufficient stabilisation and improvement in its patients for them to move back to an ordinary ward'. No reference to therapeutic objectives or methods was included in the statement. Admission to such a unit might be as a result of an incident on a ward, and, as a 'knee-jerk' response, patients would be transferred as a 'punishment' or 'to teach them a lesson'.

Over many years such units had obtained a 'macho' image which was reflected in the behaviour and approach of staff. Because of the perceived 'difficultness' or 'dangerousness' of the patients (which would be assumed, or why would they be there?), the use of a variety of methods of restraint or control was accepted. So the nurse would have no difficulty in persuading the doctor that additional medication was necessary to control behaviour and medication prescribed for the nurse to administer 'as required' might be given regularly or without due cause. Similarly, whilst policies for the control and monitoring of seclusion existed (and would be reviewed by visiting Mental Health Act Commissioners) the actual practice and use was endemic and an automatic response to any incident or potential incident. There were few signs of post-incident review by the clinical team, or attempts to establish alternative practices, as usage of seclusion was a daily occurrence. Staff were the main beneficiaries of the punitive approach with little, if any, thought being given to the impact upon mentally disordered patients either as individuals or a group. However machismo brought stresses upon staff arising from the confrontational relationship with their patients and the necessity for all nurses to conform to the culture and not to betray emotions of fear or concern.

CUSTODIAL CARE

The custodial approach to care and treatment was the most common, and was widely evident across the Special Hospitals. Custodial care was characterised by passive acceptance and, frequently, resignation to the working environment and all it represented. The need for individualised care was acknowledged and effective long-term relationships between staff and patients would be present. Sometimes these might be perceived by the outsider as excessively paternalistic or maternalistic and liable to promote institutionalisation. However there would be little enthusiasm for, or participation in, a structured approach to individualised care and treatment planning. The nurses' role was reactive, rather than proactive, and tolerant of the need for the patient to participate in 'therapy' or daily activity. However nurses would not see it as part of their role to be actively and regularly involved in the delivery of such activity. They would be bystanders and not participants in social and recreational events. Other 'visiting' professional staff, whether or not members of the ward clinical team, would be tolerated providing they were not perceived as challenging the status quo.

The adoption of a custodial approach could be an important coping mechanism for staff, and the least stressful. It reflected the introvert and over-defensive nature of the institutions and acted as a buffer against change or critical examination of traditional attitudes and practices. The hospitals had, for many years, had large training schools for psychiatric nursing and Ashworth and Rampton Hospitals had also trained nurses for the learning disabled. Broadmoor Hospital lost approval for training during the 1980s but Ashworth and Rampton Hospitals continued with their own pre-registration training schools until the advent of Project 2000 courses in the early 1990s. For many years training experience had largely been obtained within the hospital and this situation, combined with geographical and institutional isolation and a rigid system of internal promotion, inevitably perpetuated stasis and conformity.

NURSES AS PARTICIPANTS IN THERAPY AND TREATMENT

The punitive and custodial models were, to a limited extent, modified by a small, but committed, caucus of nurses who were interested in developing a broader and more therapeutic role and model of nursing. Such nurses were present at all levels within the nursing hierarchy and they faced the extremely difficult task of not conforming to the norms of the establishment and challenging the status quo. Some tried, but finding the pressures for conformity so overwhelming, left to take up alternative employment.

In the most fruitful situations, in addition to undertaking relevant further training or academic studies, nurses learned and developed their skills alongside other professionals, particularly psychologists.

Conversely there was sometimes passive resistance or outright antagonism from others, both within nursing and from other disciplines. Territorial concerns arose as these areas of therapeutic activity were perceived as the domain of other disciplines such as psychologists or social workers. Other nurses per-

ceived such activity as getting too close to the patient and challenging the traditional 'distancing' between nurse and patient.

A STRATEGY FOR NURSING

These alternative approaches within nursing practice were, of course, not entirely discrete but their characteristics were apparent both to those working in
the hospitals and to those with responsibility for management and review of
services. Throughout the history of the hospitals there had never been an opportunity to address the nature of nursing, the implications of the secure environment for nursing practice, or the interface with psychiatric nursing practice
elsewhere. There was an immediate need, for the first time, to establish a strategy that would address these circumstances and which would create a vision for
the body of nursing within the special hospitals as a whole, as well as for each
individual nurse. Somehow the best of relevant nursing practice, both from
within and without the hospitals, needed to be harnessed and to be established
as the basis for future development.

To be of value, and to be a real driver of change, it was essential that the
strategy for nursing should set out unambiguous and measurable aims and objectives. From the outset, in order that there should be a degree of ownership, of
the final product, that is, a range of nurses was drawn from all areas of the service. During a series of workshops focusing both upon existing good practice
and future direction, a set of clear aims and objectives was distilled.

For many participating nurses this was their first opportunity to consider
the dimensions of professional nursing practice within the Special Hospitals.
For many, the whole concept of the profession of nursing was secondary to
their personal identity as providers of a 'special' public service. The notion of
nursing as a profession, of which each nurse could see themselves as a part, had
to be developed and reinforced through association with a range of positive
practical objectives and examples of good practice.

The strategic components, as they transpired, were not unique to the Special
Hospitals as they expressed aims and objectives which could have been appropriate to other nursing services both within psychiatry and more generally. This
very fact associated the nursing service in special hospitals with the wider profession, but it was the nurses themselves who had drawn these conclusions;
they were not a strategy imposed from above.

In addition, for the first time, the focus of nursing practice was to be based
upon the primacy of the patient. Whilst an obvious statement, this purpose was
diametrically different to the historical patterns within the well-established
systems of institutional care. These were almost universally focused around the
needs of staff, or the requirements of institutional organisation. Shift patterns,
mealtimes, the locking of rooms, the denial of privacy, the disregard of the value

of the patient's viewpoint or their need for self-respect all exemplified the fact that the patient came low in any order of priorities.

Nursing in Special Hospitals: A Nursing Strategy was published in 1991 and its aims and objectives were focused upon the patient in terms of respect for their rights and the need to promote dignity and self-respect. In addition, the means of promoting the best possible nursing practice through education, research and broadened experience were emphasised. The importance of nurses being much more open-minded in their thinking and practice was promoted through an emphasis upon multiprofessional teamwork and the building of links and alliances with relevant services elsewhere.

The Nursing Strategy required not only the commitment and support of nurses but also the co-operation of other disciplines. The expressed values needed to be shared and, if multidisciplinary teamwork was to be a reality, this clearly needed the support of other professions. To assist these objectives the Strategy was published and used as an opportunity for positive publicity regarding the steps being taken to improve services. Articles in the national and professional media signified the importance of the intended changes both externally and to hospital staff.

The more detailed series of objectives which created the meat on the bones of the key aims were prioritised and implemented progressively by the Directors of Nursing of each hospital. Areas of activity were targeted and the temptation to move on all fronts was strongly resisted as counter-productive. However certain objectives, which were part of the Authority's wider plans, were implemented simultaneously across all three hospitals. These key objectives were universally implemented to improve the lives of patients. They included the designation of clear responsibility for ward management, the development of the primary nurse role and the promotion of individualised treatment and care plans.

As a means of assisting and supporting these changes, two major activities were supported and promoted by the SHSA. First a review of the practice of seclusion was commissioned, along with the promotion of alternative responses. Secondly the development of comprehensive nursing care over 24 hours was planned and promoted to replace the prevailing practice which had been characterised as 'the hospital by day and the prison by night'.

THE USE OF SECLUSION

The practice of secluding patients within a single room and locking the door was highly common within all three hospitals. Seclusion might be within a room designated for the purpose or within the patient's own room. This practice was derived entirely from the culture and norms of the hospitals which had been established over many years.

Over their lifetime the use of seclusion had been constantly challenged by bodies with responsibility for the hospitals but the practice was generally not the subject of critical review by doctors or nurses.

The Mental Health Act Commission in its Fourth Biennial Report 1989–1991, expressed concerns:

> Since its establishment the Commission has been gravely concerned about the way in which seclusion is used in the Special Hospitals. There has never been a common definition of seclusion throughout the Special Hospital System nor a common seclusion policy... The Mental Health Act Code of Practice contains extensive guidance about the use of seclusion and the Commission takes the fairly straightforward approach that it is as applicable to the Special Hospitals as to other hospitals.

Whilst there were many expressed concerns regarding the use of seclusion, there was little factual information. Records were kept of seclusion incidents and statistics were collated from these records but, as future evidence was to demonstrate, this information was not all-inclusive or reliable. For example, all patients were normally locked in their room or bedroom throughout the night hours. For many this involved the degrading practice of 'slopping out' in the morning. There were many alternative practices around seclusion, depending upon the presenting circumstances, and not all were recorded. Concerns were therefore largely based upon perceptions and myth rather than solid factual evidence.

During 1990, early in the life of the SHSA, it was recognised that any attempt to review the use of seclusion must be based upon evidence about actual levels of usage, and an understanding of the dynamics around the reasons for adopting its use. Tom Mason, then a Charge Nurse at Ashworth Hospital, had already completed studies in relation to this subject and he was commissioned to develop his research.

A multiprofessional steering group was established, representative of interests and knowledge within this field both from within and without the Special Hospitals.

The group spent time visiting and talking to patients and staff. Members reviewed the literature in relation to the use of seclusion and alternative practices and received and interpreted the information arising from the commissioned research.

PRACTICES OF SECLUSION BY OTHER NAMES

An underlying principle of the work of the steering group was to comply with the Mental Health Act Code of Practice and to adhere to its guidance regarding the use of seclusion and the exploration of alternatives. Information was gathered from 71 wards in an attempt to identify seclusion 'types' and how these were defined by nurses. The Code of Practice defined seclusion as:

> The supervised enforcement of a patient alone in a room which may be locked for the protection of others from significant harm.

The research identified four main alternative practices of seclusion use in addition to the standard form of locking a patient in a room designated for the purpose. Each of these was in practice at one or more of the hospitals. All four were deemed to lie outside of the Code of Practice definition and were defined by staff in the following ways.

1. 'Security Hours'

The practice of locking patients in their single room or dormitory at night-time. For reasons of safety due to the low staffing levels at night this was considered as normal and staff working on the day shift would lock patients in before handing over to the night shift. Thereafter a patient's room would not be unlocked unless this was absolutely essential and at least one staff member would have to be called from elsewhere to ensure that two staff or more were present.

In most situations it was the practice for night staff to locate themselves outside locked dormitories. Therefore from a situation of supervision by day with a high level of staffing, patients were then locked into dormitories without any immediate supervision.

2. 'Self-Seclusion'

This practice was primarily based upon the premise that it was the patients' choice to be locked in a seclusion room or their own room. The tradition of 'self-seclusion' presented particular challenges as it was often adopted or permitted for patients who tended to inflict, or threatened to inflict, self-injury if not 'allowed into seclusion'.

3. 'Voluntary Early Beds'

This practice was based upon staff offering the opportunity, and the patient accepting, to retire early to their room or dormitory. The door would be locked and the patient perhaps occasionally observed but he or she would not return to the ward until the next morning.

4. 'Clinical Early Beds'

This practice involved the nurse recommending to the patient that they be confined to their room at hours other than at night-time. Therefore, for whatever reason, it was staff rather than patient-initiated.

Where used, these four practices were endemic, not recorded as seclusion, and assumed as part of everyday life in the hospitals. The recorded levels of the use of seclusion therefore only represented the tip of the iceberg. There was a general perception that the Code of Practice had not taken into account the particular needs and demands of the Special Hospitals and therefore they could somehow 'lie outside' of its guidance.

Even more worrying were the attempts to define the use of seclusion within terms of medical treatment. Sometimes the practice of seclusion would be combined with the administration of oral or intramuscular medication and the lines between 'treatment' and 'control' could become easily blurred. The use of seclusion would also be identified as a strategy to be adopted, as necessary, as part of a patient's individual care plan.

THE INFLUENCE OF THE ENVIRONMENT

It was apparent that many practices had arisen as a result of inappropriate ward design, including the lack of alternative space in which to manage disturbed behaviour and the ready availability, on most wards, of rooms specifically designated for seclusion. Comparison across the three hospitals made this abundantly evident. Where new or refurbished wards had been provided, with attention to lightness, airiness and adequacy of alternative spaces, the occurrence of the use of seclusion was either minimal or non-existent.

The alternative was most clearly illustrated on the ground floor of Norfolk House at Broadmoor Hospital. Before the first phase of new buildings was opened in 1991, Norfolk House was designated as the Intensive Care Unit. The ground floor contained a series of grossly inadequate single rooms, a single corridor and one day area. This unit was used for the most severely disturbed patients, but the day area was also used for visitors attending Norfolk House. Both in order to protect highly volatile patients from each other in a highly confined space, and to allow visiting to take place without disturbance, patients were confined to their rooms, not only at night-time but also for the majority or whole of the day. It was clearly difficult to criticise the staff for the way they managed the situation when they were being asked to care for such patients in totally inappropriate circumstances.

THE OPINION OF PATIENTS

The opinions of patients regarding the use of seclusion were enlightening. When interviewing patients who had been in a Special Hospital for many years the first thing which was apparent was the clarity with which they recalled periods in their life when they had been secluded and the antecedents to such events. The experience or experiences of seclusion acted as landmarks within their career as a patient and their impressions of being forcefully locked in a room by staff were not unnaturally nearly wholly negative. Therefore, whilst the clinical perception of the use of seclusion might be as part of a treatment plan, the patients' perception was contrary.

As part of the commissioned research the interviews with patients elicited the following:

- 72 per cent of patients felt that they had not received good nursing care.
- 75 per cent felt that staff placed them in seclusion because they 'have had enough of you'.
- 77 per cent felt they were neglected while they were in seclusion.
- 84 per cent felt seclusion humiliated them.
- 61 per cent believed seclusion made them distrust staff more.
- 69 per cent felt that seclusion broke confidence with staff.
- 84 per cent disagreed that associations with staff were improved after a period of seclusion.

A bare, safe room
A strong, safe gown
Just a mattress in a room
A cardboard pot
A paper cup
Have a rest!
Calm down dear
But I need to talk
I thought you would help
Alone all day
Nothing to do
Nothing to distract
My disturbed mind
Nothing to do
Nothing to see
So all I see –
I see the pain
I feel the hurt
I see the guilt
I feel the scars
The memories
So bitter
So painful

All to remind
All to torment
All bloody day
Night and week
This is a rest??
This is help???

The research demonstrated a lack of congruence between the views of staff and patients in describing the reasons for, and the process of, seclusion. The recorded reasons which nurses gave for secluding patients predominantly referred to actual or threatened violence to self or others, and lengths of periods of seclusion were normally longer when staff were involved. The other main reason for secluding related to actual or threatened self-harm, although this would clearly not be in the patient's best interests or in accordance with Code of Practice guidance.

Examples of the distance of practice from the advice of the Code of Practice included the routine seclusion of patients upon admission, maybe for a predetermined period of up to a week whilst the patient was 'assessed'. Other reports spoke of the responsibility of the nurse who had first taken the decision to seclude to also be the nurse responsible for the decision to remove from seclusion. Incredibly this might have to wait for their return from days off-duty or even a period of leave. Clearly the decision-making role of the doctor would have been totally subjugated in such situations.

THE RESPONSE

The response to this complex situation was to establish two clear objectives. First, there was a declared intention to promote alternative approaches to the care and treatment of disturbed behaviour. Second, the use of seclusion, if still felt essential within current practice, would be within the terms of the Code of Practice. We recognised from the outset that these two objectives could not be achieved without the eventual support and co-operation of the staff in all three hospitals. Therefore, a highly consultative approach to their achievement was undertaken. The steering group published a series of five consultation papers over a six-month period to April 1993. These drew upon the research evidence and were made available to patients and staff and to interested bodies concerned with psychiatric care and treatment. The papers addressed approaches to the alternative management of disturbed behaviour, the definition of seclusion and other practices of confinement, the processes of monitoring the use of seclusion and finally how resolutions to these matters could be embodied in future policy and practice.

The consultation process, with the papers acting as a focus, proved highly enlightening and there was considerable participation and interest from all quarters. The subject matter was discussed with patients in the fora of the Hospital Patient Councils and informally during visits within the hospitals. Open meetings were held as well as more focused meetings with groups of nurses and doctors. As well as being a consultative process, it was also a learning process for all involved.

By October 1993 the consultation process and commissioned research had been completed. The SHSA published its policy entitled *The Use of Seclusion and the Alternative Management of Disturbed Behaviour within the Special Hospitals*. This was accompanied by a clear policy objective stated as:

> Our objective is to promote alternative approaches to the care and treatment of disturbed behaviour and to limit the use of seclusion to exceptional circumstances.

Simultaneously a training plan was issued for adoption in each hospital, although the process itself had already raised awareness and the process of change was underway.

TEAM RESPONSIBILITY

The custodial model did not require or foster a team approach. Clinical meetings, when they took place, would generally be accepting of the need for seclusion and would not see the development of alternative practice as a key area for debate or change. No meaningful audit of the use of seclusion, and therefore discussion of trends and solutions, would occur.

As part of the wider focus upon the importance of the multidisciplinary team, the vital contribution of each of its members, and the promotion of team building, the issue of seclusion was advanced to a central position. Firstly the historical evidence was considered. On each ward consideration was given to the frequency and length of use and the promotion of alternative practices. As a result of this review a quarter of all wards (the majority at Rampton Hospital) decided that they no longer needed to use seclusion and converted rooms designated for this purpose to other uses.

The collection and review of more accurate data regarding the use of seclusion was encouraged. This data, and its use, had never been considered as appropriate material for clinical audit which had generally been medically focused – further evidence of lack of medical support and interest in the subject. Therefore the promotion of this issue within the framework of clinical audit and quality assurance enabled a multidisciplinary focus. The collected data included frequency, length of episodes, timings of observations and reviews and reasons for confinement. These, in turn, were related to gender, ethnicity and location. Therefore the practices of regular recording, analysis and feedback became routine as well as acting as a focus for monitoring activity and change in each hospital. The other practices of seclusion, which had previously remained unrecorded, were outlawed, most significantly as a result of the introduction of 24-hour therapeutic care. Therefore, for the first time, the true levels of use of seclusion were being reported.

THE POLICY ISSUES

During the course of its work, and in light of the research evidence, the steering group came to the view that it would be impractical and dangerous to immediately outlaw the use of seclusion. Firstly, 24-hour therapeutic care had not been introduced and the plan for its full introduction would take some years to achieve. Secondly, it was important that the review of, and training in, alternative practices should be sufficiently thorough to ensure that staff developed confidence in their practice without being pressurised into unprofessional solutions. Whilst both the Authority and the steering group saw the eradication of seclusion as a highly desirable outcome it was recognised that the current state of knowledge and practice would not permit it.

The conditions of seclusion were reviewed and the design of rooms to be used for this purpose was seriously considered for the first time, again based upon the principles of the Code. Heating, lighting, ventilation, seating, bedding and the means of control and observation were incorporated in these design principles. Normally, if a patient needed to be secluded, this would be in appropriate dress for the day or night.

The frequency of observation of a patient in seclusion and the medical reviews proved to be the most difficult issues in relation to the implementation of a new policy. The simple position of the steering group was that if a patient required to be secluded, this should only be when all other alternatives had failed and should no longer be perceived as a routine practice. In addition there needed to be heightened recognition that to be secluded was a profound event in a patient's life and, as such, should be treated as a serious medical emergency. The counter argument that a patient, when secluded, could be left without attention and observation was illogical as it implied that the circumstances could not have been serious enough to warrant such drastic action.

THE ALTERNATIVE MANAGEMENT OF DISTURBED BEHAVIOUR

The initial objective of consulting regarding alternatives was to create a questioning environment through which the use of seclusion would be challenged and become the exception rather than the rule. Later, with the promotion and development of alternatives, the use of seclusion would diminish and gradually be eradicated in more and more wards.

First it was essential for staff to understand and review their reactions to disturbed behaviour. Natural fear and aggressive response in the face of violent behaviour may provoke a situation to the point where seclusion is seen as the only answer. Continuing episodes may lead to social distancing and a recurring cycle.

A second consideration was the culture which dictated standard responses within an institution. Cultures organised around control and dominance, with their traditions of toughness and machismo, do not admit the presence of fear or anxiety or permit a constructively reflective approach to practice. Even though this might not dictate the attitudes and approach of all staff, the dominant response to an aggressive episode will prevail.

In particular, alternative responses had to be sought to self-harming behaviour and suicidal ideation or attempts. The needs of patients in such circumstances were for support, guidance and human contact and nurses had to learn how to provide such a supportive environment without resorting to confinement in order to simplify observation. Alternative therapeutic skills which could respond to such situations had to be developed and the team's responsibility to seek supportive solutions became paramount.

THE THERAPEUTIC ALTERNATIVES

The creation of a fulfilled life within a secure environment is not easy, but the history of institutions demonstrates that the relief of boredom and creation of purpose within individual lives will be effective in reducing disturbance and dissent.

Based upon these principles, the requirement for purposeful occupational and rehabilitative activity was re-emphasised. Such activities had for too long been provided upon the basis of perceived need or tradition. They were not related to patient need as defined within their care plans and many patients lay outside of the ambit of such activities with, consequently, unfulfilled lives. Target standards were set for the levels of provision of organised work or activity for all patients and their achievement was monitored.

In addition, the importance of social, recreational and diversional activity was stressed particularly for those patients who would traditionally not have been provided with such opportunities due to their actual or potential threat to themselves or others. Smaller facilities for the structured outlet of aggression were provided in addition to the existing gymnasia. Multi-sensorial rooms were also provided. Such rooms, through the use of specialist lighting, music and other sensory effects, provide an environment for relaxation and may be used in conjunction with alternative therapies such as aromatherapy or reflexology. Their use proved particularly useful for patients who are able to anticipate a possible episode of disturbance or inclination to self-harm.

THE ENVIRONMENTAL ALTERNATIVES

Environmental standards were set for all wards. Targets were set to reduce the maximum ward size to 20 beds, and to 12 beds where special care facilities were to be provided. Each patient, where not already the case, was to have their own room and privacy and, where able, their own key which could only be overridden by staff in an emergency.

Other target standards included the provision of alternative day and activity spaces, distinction of smoking and non-smoking areas, patient-to-staff call systems and improvements in the décor and ward environments. Newly built wards demonstrated the positive effects on behaviour of increased daylight and airiness.

THE DEVELOPMENT OF 24-HOUR THERAPEUTIC CARE – NO LONGER 'A HOSPITAL BY DAY AND A PRISON BY NIGHT'

From 1992 onwards a main objective of the SHSA was to develop care and treatment throughout 24 hours and to banish the practice of staff locking patients in their room or dormitory for the night. If this objective could be achieved it would also banish the practice of 'slopping out'. The majority of rooms did not have en suite facilities.

The plan was ambitious and expensive. Estimates for the additional costs were in the region of £8 million, by far the majority of which was to provide adequate and safe nursing staff cover. There was also an initial degree of resistance from all professions. The existing practice was accepted to such a degree that many questioned the need for change. This response was demonstrative of the degree to which a 'prison' culture remained and the concept of 'hospital' was still foreign. Ironically, planning of medium secure regional hospital secure units, mostly during the 1980s, had always ensured that ward sizes were kept low (generally never more than 15 beds) and that safe levels of staffing were provided throughout 24 hours. The concept of locking patients in their own room would not have arisen because this would automatically have been perceived as amounting to seclusion. However, although the need for continuous care and treatment was most evidently also required for patients in high security hospitals, the issue had never been addressed.

The key question arose – how could a health service for mentally disordered people, which chose to lock up its patients at night, hope to reduce the use and incidence of seclusion during the daytime? This practice did amount to seclusion and there should be no equivocation about the matter.

The concept of '24-hour therapeutic care' therefore served as the most radical and significant example of the move from prison values to a hospital ethos. It served as a direct challenge to those staff who wished to perpetuate a custodial or punitive approach and was the clearest example that the needs of the patient were the central focus of the service. The investment of money, time and resources to achieve this change also demonstrated that the change was the main priority of the service and that managers of the service were 'putting their money where their mouth was'.

The effects of the change went way beyond the provision of additional staff cover at night-time. Each ward had to review its operational policy over 24 hours. These issues were discussed at ward community meetings with patients participating in defining new house rules which would accommodate the new freedoms available. In particular, regimentation within the ward environment could be overcome with the greater opportunity for access to individual rooms over 24 hours and a generally more relaxed approach. Patients could obtain more control of their own environment and more respect from staff for their personal rights in terms of choice, privacy and dignity.

Whilst consultation regarding the use of seclusion proceeded, the plan for introducing 24-hour therapeutic care was beginning to be realised. Therefore, by the time the new policy was published in October 1993, the introductory plan was well established and the die was cast. An initial pilot scheme had been developed at Rampton Hospital and all the indications were that the change had been well received by patients and staff. The significance of the change was demonstrated by the comment of a nurse who had been working on night duty for 20 years. He said 'for the first time I have been able to sit down and have a conversation with a patient – it is wonderful!'.

The experience of the pilot was used to establish a short-list of basic standards for the full introduction of 24-hour therapeutic care. As far as was practical, patients would control access to their own room and privacy by having their own key (a facility patients had requested for themselves to ensure their own personal safety). They would have immediate access to sanitary facilities and the practice of 'slopping out' would be eradicated. Choice would be available in relation to bed-times and staff call communication systems were to be universally installed. In parallel, the gradual eradication of dormitories and introduction of single rooms for all facilitated the achievement of these standards.

Standards were also introduced to safeguard the position of staff and to eradicate some old custodial practices. Day and night staffing was integrated with internal rotation managed by each Ward Manager. Therefore patients would be familiar with the regular staff around the clock and continuity of care could be assured. Equal opportunities for the personal development and training of all staff was introduced.

Self-harming behaviour frequently took place during the night hours when patients were locked in their rooms. Such behaviour was particularly prevalent on women's wards and on occasion it became evident that the action was deliberate in order to be unlocked and to receive personal attention, perhaps in a general hospital. For patients prone to such behaviour the night hours were often the most difficult to face and with the change of practice this meant there was always a nurse to talk to and an opportunity for a cup of tea.

In terms of the life of patients and staff in special hospitals the changes were dramatic, but often the problems envisaged following introduction did not occur or were minimised. Initially the rolling out of the programme took place at Rampton Hospital. Groups of three or four wards were selected and training and preparation took place. Lessons were being learned from both staff and patients from the pilot areas and there was inevitable curiosity. For many staff the change was something they were finding very difficult to come to terms with. Throughout their careers they had accepted the patterns of control which were part of day-to-day life for themselves and their patients. These patterns were now being challenged and, most fundamentally, the changes challenged the traditional distance between nurse and patient. Giving patients more control over their lives, and placing expectations upon staff to put the needs of patients first, challenged the status quo. These fears and concerns were brought out as part of the programme of change and were largely resolved as each new ward adopted the changed practices.

Gradually Ashworth Hospital and finally Broadmoor Hospital came to accept that the changes were inevitable. Therefore the learning process initially took place between hospitals and later within each hospital as the programme of change was introduced. Adjustment was required and there were inevitably patients who decided that this was a good opportunity to stay up all night and would then have no desire to take part in activity the following day. However the solution to such responses rested in a changed relationship between staff and patients, a relationship based within a therapeutic milieu and a distance away from custodialism and punishment.

Inevitably learning will need to continue to establish the appropriate therapeutic milieu and the most effective approach to relationships within the environment of a special hospital. This learning must take place within a humanitarian framework which allows constant challenge to the status quo but does not undermine the value and lessons of experience. The introduction of 24-hour therapeutic care and the challenge to the use of seclusion serve as markers in this learning process and as a sound basis for future change.

CHAPTER 15

A Doctor's View

David Mawson

SPECIAL HOSPITALS

The Special Hospitals have never been popular places. They have never enjoyed the public sympathy, in respect of what they do, for whom they do it or in what circumstances. Those within the Special Hospitals have long been aware of the frosty attitudes that lie outside the walls, acute manifestations of which are all too apparent at times of catastrophe, such as following the escape and killing of a child by John Straffen from Broadmoor Hospital in 1952.

Public attitudes hardened yet further following the release of two other patients, Terence Iliffe and Graham Young, from Broadmoor Hospital in the early 1970s. Their subsequent offending led not only to a public outcry but also to the rapid establishment of a committee under the chairmanship of Lord Butler, which was required to address a number of issues in relation to mentally disordered offenders, notably those which related to the problems of reoffending. The resultant document is still of relevance today, and included seminal chapters on dangerousness, psychopathic disorders and the special verdict. As well as being a thoughtful discussion document it made several recommendations (such as those on the special verdict) which were to lie ignored and undisturbed for many years. So much of the report is pertinent, yet so few of its recommendations were followed up. There was one important exception at least, however, which concerned the proposal, made in 1974 in an interim report, which proposed the development of new facilities (medium secure units) which would specifically be developed to assist the decanting of the severely overcrowded Special Hospitals.

There were several reasons for the overcrowding and certain recent antecedents were relevant. First, in the early 1950s the introduction of Chlorpromazine and other antipsychotic medication signalled the real possibility of decarceration for the hordes of long-term inmates of the large county asylums (as they had been referred to in the County Asylums Act of 1808). The declining number of beds in such hospitals increased the pressure in the Special Hospitals. And, second, there was evidence of a political will to close these hospitals, or to let them run down. Enoch Powell, Minister of Health in 1961, made much of the alleged iniquity of these places in his 'Brooding water towers' speech. These large psychiatric hospitals were developed slowly, their legal origin the County Asylums Act of 1808. By late Victorian times there were many of them, often accommodating over 1000 patients, sometimes in what we would now consider highly inappropriate circumstances. These large communities of staff and patients were initially at some distance from the population they served until the sprawl of urban development started to engulf them. Often set in large, wooded grounds, many had tall water towers which heralded one's approach to such a hospital, and these became symbolic of the deficiencies they were felt to represent.

Slowly but surely, already evident in the early 1970s, there was a gradual reduction in the size of the large county psychiatric hospitals. As that happened patients were moved on to less supervised circumstances, perhaps in some cases to quite inappropriate community placements where deteriorating behaviour inevitably followed hard on the heels of a relapse in mental state.

Some of them offended, and were either disposed of by sentencing to prison, or were returned to hospital within the provisions of Section 60 of the Mental Health Act of 1959. Of these some will have gone to one of the then four Special Hospitals: Broadmoor, Rampton, Moss Side and Park Lane. The gradual closure or run-down of local psychiatric hospitals was not matched with an increase in alternative community resources or more suitable hospital accommodation. Baby went out with the bath water, and the four hospitals groaned with their heavy loads. Between 1958 and 1970 the three hospitals (Park Lane had not yet been built) housed more than 2150 patients, and reached a peak of about 2400 in 1974. In the following decade the number gradually fell to about 1650. Park Lane's first 100 admissions were all from Broadmoor, with one exception, a major contribution to reducing overcrowding in the Crowthorne site, although there was still a long way to go.

With hindsight one can see that the Special Hospitals were bound to be subject to radical managerial change in due course. So much was changing from the 1970s and the Butler report and the circumstances from which it arose were emblematic of what was to follow.

Public attitudes were hardening, fed with a growing, often prurient, interest of the media. Medical supremacy was being challenged, not only among other clinicians within psychiatry, but also from outside the profession. Larry Gostin's *A Human Condition* (1975) heralded a new climate of criticism of psychiatric practice, particularly in relation to the detained patient, and a number of critical watchdog organisations, such as MIND, found their feet.

At the same time many hospitals were being criticised for the care of their patients. A number of reports spoke of brutalisation of patients by staff who were weakly led by a remote management structure. By the end of the 1970s there had been in excess of 18 such reports. The hospitals, which may have enjoyed a sense of immunity from public appraisal up until then, now reeled under the critical glare of adverse publicity.

The Special Hospitals joined the process in 1980 when Rampton Hospital was criticised in the Yorkshire Television production, 'The Secret Hospital'. The Boynton report that soon followed told of antiquated practice, of an aggressive, sometimes brutal regime, and, again, weakness of management. A lack of medical leadership was roundly criticised. Several prosecutions of nursing staff were successful and, though without conspicuous publicity, some medical staff were removed or relocated.

Meanwhile the Department of Health kept its collective head down, acutely conscious no doubt of the potential hazards of too confrontational a style of central management, with the risks that attended a moment of injudicious decisiveness of the kind that would challenge the status quo. The Department's 'inside story' of the decade that led up to 1989 has yet to be told and the following comments are necessarily personal, even partisan, and undoubtedly incomplete. Yet for many of us close to the Special Hospitals during the 1980s it must have been apparent that the Department was not willing to address the principle and long-standing blemish of the Special Hospitals: the Prison Officers Association (POA). A government that had fearlessly taken on the seamen, the miners and other intransigent unions, and had been willing to pass unpopular industrial relations legislation, was nevertheless not prepared to face the POA with the same enthusiasm.

The links within the POA nationally, with their strong hold on the operation of the prisons, were far closer to the members of the unions in the Special Hospitals than they are today, and perhaps it was feared that a sneeze in the Special Hospitals could have led to pneumonia in the prison system.

In November 1987 the management of Moss Side Hospital suspended a nurse when a number of patients said he had not once, but twice within a few days, hit a patient on a ward. The local POA was incensed that management had suspended a nurse in such circumstances, insisting suspension had never happened before. They balloted for industrial action, and kept closely in touch with their lawyers and the POA's National Executives. Local managers were concerned at the angry climate of the hospital and kept the Department of Health closely informed, and were heartened by the supportive noises coming from London.

Industrial action was favoured by the membership and took the form of a lock-in of all patients (about 284) who were in effect secluded for all but three hours a day during the ten-day action. Hate mail flowed to management;

threats and intimidation of nurses who dissented were reported. An escalation of the action locally was in the air, and the strident interest and involvement of National Executive officials signalled the possibility of supportive industrial action elsewhere. The Department was in frequent daily contact with local management, anxious that a resolution to the industrial relations impasse be achieved to end the flurry of critical publicity, among other things. The Mental Health Act Commission glided silently through the hospital, in a manner reminiscent of the ghost of Lady Jane Grey, and took no public stand on the dispute while regretting its consequences for the patients. The impasse was ended when an 'independent inquiry' was set up at the Department of Health, attended by representatives of both the local and national POA, though not local managers. Their action in the suspension of the nurse was found wanting, and he was returned to the hospital to non-nursing duties. An opportunity had been lost.

Early in 1988 all of the Special Hospitals' local managers were called to the Department to discuss the problem of complaints investigations, and it was revealed that no agreement had been achieved since 1979 as to how complaints would be investigated. The POA had always resisted management's claim to be allowed to investigate complaints of a potentially 'criminal' nature (such as allegations of assault), insisting they should be passed to the police. If the police failed to establish a good enough case for prosecution (which was almost invariably the case, largely on the basis that other patients were not felt to be credible witnesses) then the issue was returned to local management. The POA would now state that further local investigation was unfair as it constituted 'double jeopardy' for those alleged to have done something wrong. Any attempt to question the person led to the accompanying official advising him not to answer. This absurd state of affairs came to an end only during the tenure of the Special Hospitals Services Authority (SHSA), when at last complaints were investigated more robustly, a procedure was laid down, and outside investigators were brought in. The events of November 1987 would have been very different two or more years later.

A NEW ERA

The arrival of new management arrangements in the autumn of 1989 received a mixed reaction among the clinicians, especially the doctors. Some disdain for the way the Medical Directors (and others) of all four hospitals were made redundant by the Department of Health, and far greater concern at yet another change, were tempered with the prospect of the possibility of a more closely involved central management and separation from what some saw as the ineffective 'dead hand' of the Department. There were local concerns for each site. Ashworth Hospital, for example, had considerable reservations, to say the least, about the amalgamation of two hospitals with two distinct cultures and patient groups on a very large site.

Each hospital's lead doctor was now the Director of Medical Services, a much reduced role in terms of authority and power, but perhaps not much less in terms of accountability for clinical matters. The new role was to continue the ever important tasks of recruitment and other medical personnel issues, and advice to the new expanded management teams, as well as other locally and historically determined tasks, but its diminished authority led some to see the change as like the difference between headmaster and head prefect. Nevertheless, the local general managers were now empowered as the hospitals' management had not been for many years. Accountability was seasoned with authority and influence.

Centrally, a new role was created in the form of the Head of Medical Services, a post held in the first five years by Pamela Taylor. Her contribution was significant, and during her tenure chairs were established at Ashworth and Broadmoor Hospitals; before the end of the life of the SHSA she had taken the chair post at Broadmoor. New developments in research and training, and an increase in the number of trainees, visiting professionals and teaching occasions were evident.

The number of consultants also showed a healthy increase, more of whom held joint academic appointment than at any previous time, and these new doctors had usually been comprehensively trained in forensic psychiatry in one of the various rotations. The case-loads of many consultants fell, although in each of the three sites there remained a number with case-loads of over 40, and a few with much higher numbers. This is still the case.

Although the issue is dealt with elsewhere, one positive development enjoyed by the medical staff, which will not be appreciated fully by the newly appointed, was the lessening of the oppressiveness of the small but powerful core membership of the POA. Early in the era of the SHSA several significant issues were 'won' by management, and other nursing unions, carriers of a different culture, gained ground. The former tendency to reach for what one POA Chairman called 'my old friend, the ballot box' now rarely showed itself. But the union's influence, though lessened, still remains and Elaine Murphy's recent call for de-recognition of the union in the three hospitals (Murphy 1997) deserves the support of the profession.

DEMANDS, CONSTRAINTS AND CHOICES

The word 'demand' has at least two major connotations: that which is required, obligatory; and that which is demanding, perhaps stressful. The Special Hospital doctor's life contains ingredients of both these themes.

The obligatory element is clearly manifest in much of the report work: provision of annual statutory reports on patients for the Home Office, reports for Mental Health Review Tribunals, outside assessments, Section 117 meetings and the Care Programme Approach, and the plethora of other time-limited reports or responses that have proliferated in the last few years. A greater emphasis on well-documented treatment planning, patient involvement and multidisciplinary input, with identification of goals (or identified problems), interventions and anticipated outcomes, became *de rigueur* well before the demise of the SHSA in April 1996. Similarly a proliferation of inquiries and complaints, often externally driven, have added to the burden, as it is sometimes perceived, of the Special Hospital doctor. These enquiries usually carry a specified time-scale response, not least when litigation seems likely. In their 1995 review the SHSA reported that there were 1737 complaints registered at the three sites, of which 395 were eventually upheld. Complaints about medical care and services comprised 8 per cent (about 139) of the total.

These demands have increased. This is not solely attributable to the SHSA, though it is true that the Authority sought to improve the hospital's response to patients' needs, and to be in a position to demonstrate and monitor it. However, in the process, some clinicians have come to maintain that their clinical time is inappropriately taken up with matters of this kind, often at the expense of face-to-face time with the patients, and the staff who care for them.

The other sort of demand is different, and takes two main forms. It transcends the era of any supervisory authority. The first form relates to the content of the history and activities of the patient population. While this is self-evident one notes that many will minimise its significance and perhaps do so at their own peril. The cheerful badinage of the profession, and not only doctors, within forensic psychiatry bears testimony to the varied attempts made by us all to distance ourselves from the sheer tragic senselessness of the offences of some of our patients, and the effects of these on so many others.

A young man killed his mother, believing she was involved with a terrorist organisation, repeatedly stabbing her. He was transferred to a Special Hospital as an emergency, having become highly disturbed on remand. Within a short time he was making a good but partial recovery. Less than three months after the offence he was playing snooker on the admission ward with another patient. He saw me watching him from the nurse's station and interrupted the game to come and talk to me. The door of the office opened and he said 'Maybe I did not kill her. Perhaps it was someone else'. There was a slight pause. 'It's worth thinking about, doc.' He left before comment was made.

Two other individuals come to mind. Both had killed all their children, and one of them had also killed his wife. The latter had done so when suffering from a paranoid psychosis, and made a full recovery after a year or so, now to be confronted with the guilt and sadness he felt for what he had done. He had previously been 'protected' by persecutory delusions in which he believed he had saved them from torture. Now much better, he contemplated suicide often, but he denied himself this, fearing what his victims would say to him when he met them in the hereafter. The other, a cold and very large man, blamed his wife for the children's deaths and saw his execution of them as just retribution for her own actions.

The catalogue of misery that precedes a patient's 'index offence' (a term itself redolent with a sense of detachment) may be awesome. So few patients graduate to the Special Hospitals without themselves having been subject to neglect, abuse and degradation, prior to the events that promote them to care in high security. As inpatients these issues are addressed, but the problems are not over. The abused can themselves offer abuse to others, and within the hospitals acts of major violence punctuate the gloom, themselves carrying a toll for all those in the vicinity.

The other stressful demand facing clinicians throughout psychiatry as a whole, though no less within the three hospitals, is the inquiry. Each hospital has had several, arising in a range of circumstances, such as the death of a patient following restraint and forcible injection; absconsion and escape; the homicide of a patient; a hostage-taking; a cluster of suicides. In a number of inquiries, often protracted and publicised, individuals were named and criticised, including some of the medical staff. Of all the inquiries, the most detailed and widely promulgated was the Ashworth Inquiry, evidence for which was taken in a lengthy hearing in Liverpool from September 1991. More than 80 witnesses gave evidence to the panel of four, chaired by (now Sir) Louis Blom-Cooper, regarding four major complaints of untoward incidents, and a number of lesser matters. The former included allegations of physical assaults, sexual assault on a female patient, and the sudden death of a patient in seclusion. In their extensive report (Blom-Cooper *et al.* 1992) the panel describe evidence of a culture of denigration of patients, physical and mental bullying by staff, overt racism and a poor quality of care. Excessive use of seclusion, poor clinical teamwork, and intimidation of members of the Royal College of Nursing by various means were described. Local management team members were criticised (and named) for their failure to deal adequately with complaints and for a lack of leadership.

The report exercised equally strong terms for the role of the Mental Health Act Commission (MHAC) in dealing with complaints, a task specified within Section 120 (1) (b) (i) and (ii) of the Mental Health Act (1983). The authors concluded that the Commission had been 'notably disengaged from the complaints system operative at the hospital', with 'marginal' engagement to the conclusion of complaints investigations: 'How the endless complaints from patients which "flowed down in streams" – to adapt the Swiftian metaphor – failed to engage the intention of the MHAC, seems to us an impropitious curiosity, explicable in parts by the exasperation of a defective complaints system in which the Commission was entangled as a kind of appellate body.' The Commission reported to the Inquiry that: 'It is apparent that the patients, on the whole, never became convinced that the MHAC could sufficiently challenge the special hospital's system so as to be effective on the patients' behalf. Perhaps there was no greater touchstone of the failure than the complaints system'. Resounding, but unattributed, criticism.

One senior academic in forensic psychiatry once told me, soon after the report's publication, that it was better to be criticised by a bad inquiry than a good one. I was grateful at the time for his remark, as I felt hurt and betrayed, if that's not too strong a phrase, by certain individuals and organisations that might have presented the Inquiry with evidence in 'mitigation'. But the glaring fact was that, the pride of those like myself not withstanding, places that purport to provide care for a highly vulnerable population – mentally disordered, compulsorily detained and with little power – should be obliged to serve the interests of such patients as best they can. Whether we like it or not, and despite the limitations and bias of an inquiry of this kind, the Ashworth Inquiry will later be remembered as having further empowered the SHSA in a way that perhaps no single Minister or collective government could possibly have done. Examples of the improvements made include the strengthening of the complaints system, and the ending of seclusion at night. (That is, patients are not confined to their rooms between 9 pm and 7 am, as they had been previously.) The issue of '24-hour therapeutic care', whereby patients are allowed free egress from their rooms at any time of night or day (subject to some qualifications), remains a contentious one within the hospitals at certain levels and the facility would, no doubt, be rescinded quickly if a breach of security were attributable to it. Nevertheless, the report gave much strength to the new Authority which came into an environment that was deeply conservative in style. If the report incurred some casualties the benefits probably far outweighed the disadvantages.

Inquiries generally find little favour with psychiatrists, especially those on the receiving end. They can be the 'pay-off' for years of dealing with ungrateful patients in a less than perfect setting, on behalf of a society that at times seems neither to understand nor care. It has been argued (Muijen 1997) that inquiries are costly, and that the current system of inquiry is damaging to everyone, adding little to our knowledge of what can and does go wrong. Muijen says that the system of inquiry should involve scrutiny of the issues by an authoritative body, with the use of panel inquiries only in exceptional cases. In response Grounds (1997) agreed that improvements were required, but felt that both the public and psychiatry need to learn from inquiries. And, above all, the families of the bereaved, in the case of a homicide inquiry, need to know what happened and to have confidence that any mistakes made would not be repeated.

Constraints on the doctors are rather more obvious. Whereas, prior to 1989, a panel at the DHSS had to agree a recommended admission to, say, Broadmoor Hospital, it now became necessary to submit a report to the hospital-based admissions panel. The panel comprised a multidisciplinary group, usually chaired by the Medical Director. Reports recommending admission outlined the details of the personal and family background history of the patient, the evidence of the mental disorder and an assessment of the dangerousness of that patient. The test of the latter was whether, if at large, the patient would pose a grave and immediate danger to members of the public, either individually or collectively. If this test was not satisfied a bed would not be offered. If the panel agreed the recommendation – and it was usually so – the patient would be admitted, subject to the agreement of the court or pertinent others, and after treatment, perhaps many years later, a patient might be recommended for discharge or transfer. This would now involve the Home Office (in 80 per cent of cases), a receiving hospital or community placement, and between those two processes the patient's progress might often be at the whim of bed availability, and other factors, and thus could be lost to the supervision of the consultant who initiated admission.

Unlike the consultant in most of the existing secure units, the Special Hospital consultant has little influence on the progress of the patient he or she seeks to admit. While admittedly long time-scales are involved for many of these, this nevertheless serves to emphasise the sense of powerlessness of the doctors in the march of patient care. At least one hospital's consultants attempted a 'cradle to the grave' policy, whereby the admitting consultant sought to have responsibility for the patients he or she admitted all the way through the hospital. Inevitably this led to having patients on many wards, perhaps six or seven, with the consequent fragmentation of multidisciplinary team-working, and the reduction of the impact of clinicians, other than nurses, on ward culture.

Colleagues in medium secure units enjoy greater freedom of clinical practice and diversity of experience than their Special Hospital counterparts. Their smaller inpatient case-loads are often supported by trainees in forensic psychiatry, by no means the norm in a high security hospital, allowing them to do work in different settings such as prisons, courts and with other services, such as probation. Joint appointments at consultant level between secure units and the special hospitals are very rare, and the secure unit doctors admit reluctance to engage in work in a system they consider too large, isolated and institutional. The lack of professional autonomy and the perception of heavier management style further deters their engagement. These issues also influence recruitment, although the traditionally heavier case-loads in Special Hospitals are perhaps the greatest obstacle to recruitment.

Choices are nowadays more available. Joint academic appointments are encouraged and their number is increasing, allowing for the few a greater diversity of work and research or training opportunities. Such consultants have generally small, manageable case-loads, with the interest and support of trainees. But these posts are the exception, and too many consultants continue to have 40 patients, and a few even more. Unless radical measures are taken to reduce the size of the hospitals' populations (it is well established that several hundred patients only require lesser security) there must be a significant increase in the number of doctors employed at each site. Furthermore, the three hospitals should be unshackled from the constraints of the current pay structure.

PSYCHOPATHIC DISORDER

Few topics engender such fevered debate among clinicians in special hospitals as the treatment of the 'psychopath'. Such discussions start evenly enough. Common ground is acknowledged: that 'psychopathic disorder' is a medico-legal device; that current classifications leave much to be desired; and that its origins are multi-factorial, and its manifestations protean. Nor are the clinical features and potential risks posed by a particular individual with personality disorder usually a major source of dispute (though this is not always the case when discharge is being considered, say, at a Mental Health Review Tribunal).

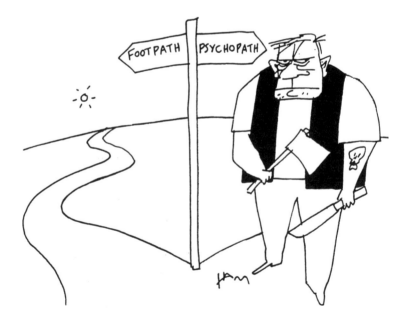

Figure 15.1 Cartoon by Ham Khan
Source: The Observer

Perhaps the most heat is reserved for two main areas. First, are such persons 'treatable', both within the legal definition and from a clinical point of view? And, second, if they are (or may be) when should they get that treatment?

The legal issue of treatability can be dispatched quickly. For someone with psychopathic disorder the responsible medical officer has to show at the time of detention that the patient is treatable, that the proposed treatment will alleviate the condition or prevent further deterioration, neither of which notions are defined, but it is hard to see how most patients could fail to satisfy the last criterion. On occasion the consultant will report to a tribunal that a patient remains dangerous but is untreatable, anticipating that failure to be treatable will lead to a patient's discharge, perhaps after a seemingly fruitless decade or two in hospital. Such a recommendation, while understandable in that a chronically 'stuck' patient can be very frustrating and demoralising, may be unwise to the point of recklessness in some cases. However, following what is known as the Andrews case (not concerning a Special Hospital patient), the tribunal is not obliged to discharge a patient who is considered untreatable.

Treatability from a clinical point of view is more problematic. Research in this field is fraught with problems, but some studies suggest cautious optimism while others give equivocal or negative results (helpful reviews include those of Tyrer and Stein 1993, and Dolan and Coid 1993). And what can the Special Hospitals do for such patients? My own view, held since I first worked in a Special Hospital over 15 years ago (Mawson 1983), is not very much. True, some patients do benefit from time and access to a range of therapeutic and other opportunities, but it is very difficult indeed to know which ones will.

And the cost of failure is high, both for the patient and the institutions. In view of the fact that some might benefit, though which was uncertain, my preference was to offer treatment to such people on a transfer direction (that is, moving a sentenced prisoner to hospital, rather than having a hospital order from the court at the time of sentencing). This would allow research and treatment on a larger number of patients, a far more cost-effective exercise. Instead of having one patient for 20 years (who would presumably be a treatment failure) one could treat, say, ten patients for two years each, a number of whom might benefit. Better this way by far, in my view, than admitting a patient on a hospital order who proves inaccessible to all that is offered, only to become a major management problem or a deeply institutionalised mainstay of the hospital shop. Neither outcome is good for the patient or the hospitals, least of all when all three have a waiting list for admission.

Some will maintain that treatability can be adequately assessed by means of the interim order, which allows patients to be assessed for up to six months in hospital while on remand and before sentencing. Apart from the fact that this is the most expensive investigation in medicine (costing about £40,000 at current prices), it is not the best time and means to accurately predict response to treatment. The implications for subsequently recommending a hospital order to the court are huge, and Grounds (1987) thoughtfully outlined the six questions he felt were critical to the issue:

o Do such offenders have a definite mental disorder?

o What constitutes treatment?

o Who is 'treatable'?

o Is treatment effective?

o Does psychological change imply reduced risk of offending?

o Is indeterminate sentencing for treatment a fair exchange for sentencing based on justice?

He felt the evidence at each stage was lacking, a view with which I fully concur. These questions, and no doubt many others critical to the treatment of such patients in high security hospitals, will doubtless be a substantial component of the review about to get underway at Ashworth Hospital at the time of writing.

REFERENCES

Blom-Cooper, L. *et al.* (1992) *Report of the Committee of Inquiry into Complaints about Ashworth Hospital.* HMSO Cm 2028–I and II.

Dolan, B. and Coid, J. (1993) *Psychopathic and Antisocial Personality Disorders – Treatment and Research Issues.* London: Gaskell.

Gostin, L.O. (1975) *A Human Condition: The Law Relating to Mentally Abnormal Offenders: Observations, Analysis and Proposals for Reform.* Vol.2. London: MIND.

Grounds, A.T. (1987) 'Detention of "psychopathic disorder" patients in special hospitals: critical issues.' *British Journal of Psychiatry 151,* 474–478.

Grounds, A.T. (1997) 'Commentary on "Inquiries, who needs them"' *Psychiatric Bulletin 21, 3,* 133–134.

Mawson, D.C. (1983) '"Psychopaths" in special hospitals.' *Bulletin of the Royal College of Psychiatrists 7,* 178–181.

Muijen, M. (1997) 'Inquiries, who needs them?' *Psychiatric Bulletin 21, 3,* 132–133.

Murphy, E. (1977) 'The future of Britain's high security hospitals.' *British Medical Journal 314,* 1292–1293.

Tyrer, P. and Stein, G. (1993) *Personality Disorder Reviewed.* London: Gaskell.

CASES CITED

R v Cannons Park Mental Health Review Tribunal [1993] (Ex parte A). United Kingdom.

CHAPTER 16

Working Together

Improving Care

Jane Mackenzie

INTRODUCTION

Broadmoor Hospital in the late 1960s was not an environment where terms such as 'shared professional values', 'professional collaboration', 'sensitivity to patient needs', 'clinical leadership' or 'individualised care and treatment planning', 'skilled assessment' would have been used in relation to multidisciplinary teams, or their work. Yet in 1997 these are some of the phrases used in a letter that I wrote to a multidisciplinary team, just after I'd attended one of their weekly ward meetings. I had been invited to the meeting and been extremely impressed with the professionalism, the caring attitude, the way every member of the team respected each other and demonstrably valued each other's contribution to the review of the patients' care and treatment plans. There was a high degree of skills and knowledge demonstrated by the team and real collaboration was evident. The patient was warmly welcomed by the team and treated with extreme sensitivity. The varying assessments carried out by every member of the team had been made available to the patient some time before the meeting and he had been asked if he agreed with the assessment they had made. The patient was also encouraged to present his own summary of events, both at the meeting and as a written record. The whole experience contrasted starkly with recollections of my first attendance at a 'case conference' as a student nurse at Broadmoor Hospital in 1968.

As one of eight first-year student nurses, I was invited to attend a patient's case conference as part of our studies. The male consultant psychiatrist, although small in stature, presented an awesome and commanding figure. Standing in the middle of a large meeting room, he alone presented the patient's case history in a 'lecture' style – the 'invited' guests merely listened. The patient was brought into the conference and appeared to have had no prior warning about the conference, or what was expected of him. He appeared overwhelmed by the large group, was not offered a chair on which to sit, and looked anxious and uncomfortable. He must have felt, as I did, from the barrage of questions insensitively asked, that he was being put 'on trial' for his index offence. When we were given the opportunity to ask questions, as an enthusiastic student nurse, I naively asked a question that I cannot quite recall, but I know it reflected a hint of a challenge! What I can remember, as if it was yesterday, was being made to feel like a three-year-old who had just been very naughty! The consultant psychiatrist made it very clear that he thought it was a pretty stupid question and cynically asked about the length of time I had been in training, and what academic qualifications were required for student nurses training these days; he did not answer my question! I still recall being unable to lift my eyes up from the floor, feeling acutely embarrassed and seeing through blurred and watery eyes, a pair of white socks on the feet of this otherwise very elegantly dressed man. This introduced an element of repressed hysteria, and I was not quite sure whether I would laugh or cry; I did neither. After what seemed like forever, I was allowed to 'slink' back into oblivion. I came out of that room with a fierce determination to pursue the education, the knowledge and confidence needed, not just to contribute to the provision of care and treatment of people who have serious and enduring mental illness, but to be able to challenge and ultimately change the 'caring' profession I had just entered. These thoughts were with me the day I graduated with a Masters Degree from Birmingham University in 1995, and I wished that the consultant, white socks and all, could have been there!

This chapter describes some of the developments and influences between that first multidisciplinary meeting in 1968 and a recent meeting I attended in 1997, that have contributed to the radical changes in the way multidisciplinary teams provide care and treatment for patients at Broadmoor Hospital.

'England does not like Coalitions' (Disraeli, 1807–1895)

This political statement made almost a century ago may well have summed up the philosophy of multiprofessional clinical teams at that time and well on into this century. Despite the introduction of the NHS in 1946 the anticipated co-operation between health care services did not occur for many years. Until very recently, barriers have remained within the NHS between members of various mental health professions who have provided health care, often in isolation and rarely collaboratively. At Broadmoor Hospital, the picture reflected that of the mainstream NHS with the additional difficulties of providing health care in a secure environment with a deeply embedded culture, not always conducive to professional or harmonious team-working. The past decade has seen the removal of many of the barriers individual professions tend to surround themselves with, and an emphasis on true multidisciplinary teamwork.

The term 'collaboration' is often used to describe the ideal team, summing up a vision of total harmony and a group of people pulling together. The Oxford Dictionary definition of 'collaboration', however, has a different connotation:

Collaboration: 'to co-operate traitorously with an enemy'

This definition of collaboration may well have been the thinking of the professionals as they started to work together in teams.

BACKGROUND

Historically, the care and treatment provided by professionals in Special Hospitals was not too different from any conventional psychiatric establishment up until the late 1960s, where the culture was one of control and containment and where multidisciplinary teams did not exist. Prior to the introduction of registered training for nurses, 'attendants', who were in the main untrained and unskilled, struggled to provide care for patients, who were extremely violent and dangerous, under the 'direction' of the Responsible Medical Officer. There was little support available from other services; other disciplines at that time were rarely, if ever, involved.

The hospital 'administrator' provided some support and services to patients, now normally carried out by the social work and finance departments. Treatment consisted mainly of medication, seclusion and workshops consisting of industrial/occupational therapy. At Broadmoor Hospital, as in other establishments, RMOs, (now called Consultant Forensic Psychiatrists), often had excessively large case-loads (up to 200 patients) and they would normally only discuss patients' care and treatment, with the Sister or Charge Nurse of the ward.

Because of their heavy case-loads, the psychiatrists on the whole were only able to spend a minimal amount of time on each ward, dealing with the most difficult patients and priority problems. They were, therefore, quite content for the day-to-day management and care provision on the wards to be carried out by the Ward Sister/Charge Nurse, who often ruled the patients and staff with a rod of iron to maintain a 'steady' status. There were no structured assessments, no care or treatment planning and there was no formal evaluation of progress, other than an annual case conference, which was, as far as I could see, necessary to continue the patient's detention order and contribute to the training of staff. Challenging practices and/or attitudes was not encouraged, and multidisciplinary teamwork was not promoted, encouraged or supported in any way. The role of the consultant remained autocratic and autonomous for many years, with little evidence of participation in patient care from other disciplines. When other professions began to expand within the hospital, their views and contributions were kept very much on the periphery and collaborative approaches were, on the whole, actively discouraged. This restricted their roles and prevented them asserting their professional values and responsibilities. Psychologists tended to retreat into research and respond to the occasional referral for a psychological assessment. Social workers' main role was to visit patients' families, and provide a social history based on this. None of these key professions were considered as members of the team and they were on the whole treated with suspicion and disdain. Poor teamwork, communications and treatment planning have often been highlighted in inquiries and reports into care and treatment within Special Hospitals.

The concept of patient participation and involvement was not on the agenda at all!

Nurses and other disciplines were not encouraged to speak to Consultant Forensic Psychiatrists; communication continued to be held mainly between them and the Ward Sister or Charge Nurse of the ward.

This doctor/nurse power-base dominated the treatment philosophy and, I believe, prevented the development of multidisciplinary teamwork and treatment planning for many years.

DEFINING MULTIDISCIPLINARY TEAMS

In 1979, the Royal Commission on the National Health Service defined a multidisciplinary team as 'a group of colleagues acknowledging a common involvement in the care and treatment of a particular patient'. Collegial teams are those in which members make decisions, using a consensus management style, and are differentiated by hierarchy. Campbell-Heider and Pollock (1987) defined collegiality as 'interdependent practice between physicians and nurses', and suggest that while doctors exercise most authority, nurses possess great informal power. Again the emphasis has traditionally been on the nurse/doctor input to the team. It is only recently that multidisciplinary teams are beginning to explore their own definitions of multidisciplinary teamwork and what constitutes a successful team. Team-working practices and agreeing standards within Clinical Audit and Standard Setting projects are currently supporting clinical teams to focus on areas for change and improvement in clinical care and practice. It is also notably evident that a less autocratic style of consultant forensic psychiatrist is emerging that welcomes multiprofessional participation and involvement and encourages decisions using a 'consensus management style'.

CHANGES AND INFLUENCES

Unfortunately, there has been little research into multidisciplinary teamwork within Special Hospitals. The development of multidisciplinary teams and treatment planning has not been well documented and is therefore difficult to evaluate.

Professional Accountability and Education

Throughout the past three decades, codes of professional practice and conduct and focused education programmes have been initiated, by various professions, that have focused clearly on a multidisciplinary team approach, but enabled each profession to maintain and promote their own individual accountability. Professional individual accountability also, however, had its down side, as it also meant that other disciplines could no longer 'conveniently' off-load responsibility and blame medical staff for clinical errors and poor practice. Some people found this concept and the inherent responsibilities within that, quite difficult to accept.

Political, Trade Union and Social Influences

The role of the Prison Officers' Association (POA) within the Special Hospitals was very powerful and continued to promote the custodial perspective for many years. There was little emphasis on a therapeutic or multiprofessional approach. This culture predominated in the 1960s and 1970s, and the likelihood of creating a climate where teams of professionals would collaboratively provide high standards of care and treatment to patients within a high security environment seemed remote. In recent years, a far more collaborative partnership between managers, clinicians and the Prison Officers' Association has resulted in an environment where a more professional and therapeutic approach has been encouraged and clinical team-working seen as an essential part of the delivery of care. This approach reflected the leadership styles of the Special Hospitals Service Authority (SHSA) and the Broadmoor Hospital management team, who, despite many hurdles, were proactive and relentless in developing healthy, open and honest relationships with the POA. This collaboration enabled the creation of an agenda that incorporated improved professional practice and a more harmonious team approach to care.

The distant and remote management style of the Home Office and the Department of Health did little to demonstrate a clear direction for the Special Hospitals. There was little focus on the development of professional and clinical skills and practice that would underpin the development of multidisciplinary teamwork. Changes in authority to the Special Hospitals Service Authority (SHSA), in 1989, accelerated the development of multidisciplinary teamwork and treatment planning, through the setting of clear objectives and the implementation of a Patients' Charter, focusing clearly on multidisciplinary teamwork and outlining a contract for services that identified multidisciplinary standards explicitly. These standards continued to be regularly monitored and analysed and improvements made, where relevant.

Frameworks for Multidisciplinary Teamwork/Treatment Planning

It is essential that, to work effectively, multidisciplinary teams discuss and agree their core values and beliefs about what they are there to do, for their patient group.

In order to work to a shared purpose it is essential that multidisciplinary teams formally define and agree a shared philosophy and clarify all team members' roles within that.

Although in the 1970s the philosophy of multidisciplinary teamwork and treatment planning had begun to develop and relationships were improving between the varying disciplines, teamwork and treatment planning remained unstructured and fragmented. Without clear and explicit standards, working practices of multidisciplinary teams remained *ad hoc* for some time. I believe that the introduction of the Nursing Process at Broadmoor Hospital in 1985 inadvertently contributed a great deal to the development of the professional multidisciplinary teamwork and treatment planning we see today. This systematic approach to planning nursing care, although initially creating professional difficulties within the team, I believe helped establish the basis for the structured approaches to the planning of care/treatment planning we have in place today.

'Give us the tools and we'll finish the job' (Churchill, 1941)

The following standards have been introduced and have provided a focus with which multidisciplinary teams can plan and review their activities.

Clear standards for multidisciplinary treatment planning have been initiated for all clinical teams and are regularly monitored:

- A standardised multidisciplinary treatment planning framework, comprising a problem/needs assessment, a plan, agreed goals, evaluation and outcomes, has been developed, based on contract standards, and is used by each clinical team.

- Treatment plans are reviewed by all members of the clinical team led by the consultant, within six months of admission.

- The date for review of the treatment plan is agreed with the patient and recorded.

- Major treatment plan reviews take place at agreed intervals of no longer than 12 months.

These standards are regularly monitored through the process of clinical audit and other monitoring activities.

Patients' Participation/involvement

Core standards have been agreed that clearly state that the patient must be involved in their care and treatment planning. Measurement techniques used to monitor achievements in this area incorporate numerous methods, for example, seeking patients' views and retrospective record audits of treatment plans.

WHAT HAVE WE LEARNED ABOUT WORKING TOGETHER?

Team-Building Activities

Formalised team-building activities for multidisciplinary teams have been extensively used in an effort to break down 'professional barriers' and have helped to focus on collaboration, relationships and communications within the team.

Project Groups

Demonstrable improvements can be observed in the way different professionals work together and have occurred almost as a secondary 'spin-off', when multidisciplinary teams have come together to focus on a particular project such as: a Seclusion Monitoring and Review Group (SMARG), Clinical Audit Committee, Investors in People Group.

Very often, teams working on a project will develop a sense of team spirit and collaboration naturally, as the group share a common objective. Agreeing and achieving positive outcomes and developing effective relationships with patients, has also been identified as a rewarding and collaborative experience for teams. There is a clear lesson to be learned about successful teams from these activities.

The Medical Model

Difficulties have been and are still sometimes experienced with the medical model of care, so often autocratic in its provision. Some members of the medical profession have found it difficult to embrace this changing 'collaborative' philosophy, reflecting a shifting power-base.

Many consultants, however, have embraced the changing philosophy, and have welcomed the challenges and opportunities the changes have brought.

Chairmanship/Leadership

The principles and importance of good leadership and team management to develop effective teams have been well documented. The successful and effective multidisciplinary team will inevitably possess a skilled and charismatic leader, who will be able to nurture and develop the team, bringing together the available skills and qualities of the members to help to achieve its aims.

The difficulties of translating the principles of leadership into practice within a clinical team cannot be understated. It is important first to establish who 'the leader' is. The role of the leader of the multidisciplinary team has traditionally fallen to the Consultant Forensic Psychiatrist, whose role is clearly defined within the Mental Health Act as being responsible for the care and treatment of patients in their care. This can create conflicting roles and professional rivalries within the team.

Numerous models of teamwork have been identified in recent years; however, successful teamwork is not easily achieved. As an example of this, a system of collaborative care planning was developed in general and primary health care settings and seen as 'the way forward'. It was introduced into Broadmoor Hospital as a pilot project in 1994. Although some clinical teams were enthusiastic about this model of multidisciplinary teamwork and treatment planning, it was not successful. The pilot study was aborted, after a great many people had invested a great deal of money, time and enthusiasm. The key reasons for its failure to be implemented throughout the hospital were, I believe, the following two reasons:

1. The system had been developed from a different service and was not easily modified to reflect our particular service.

2. Strong personalities and conflicts about leadership and decision making within the team, together with lack of clarity and understanding of each other's roles within the team, did little to promote the harmonious working relationships required for its success. Professional conflicts and the struggle for power within the team detracted from the main objective, and what should have provided an excellent framework for multidisciplinary working failed to succeed.

Monitoring and Evaluation

The introduction by the Special Hospitals Service Authority (SHSA), of clearly defined standards within a service level agreement has enabled us as a hospital to focus on quality monitoring programmes, where explicit criteria relevant to multidisciplinary teamwork/treatment planning are measured on a regular basis.

Patients' Charters

A Patients' Charter audit has been developed, reflecting the NHS Patients' Charter and the more recently introduced Department of Health Mental

Health Service NHS Charter, and also reflecting teamwork/treatment planning.

Clinical Audit Projects

The hospital has a comprehensive clinical audit programme facilitated by a clinical audit team. Organisational standards in areas that include multidisciplinary teamworking/treatment planning are regularly audited. Locally developed standards are agreed by individual multidisciplinary teams and supported through the clinical audit programme.

Care Programme Approach

The Care Programme Approach (CPA) was introduced at Broadmoor Hospital in 1998. An audit, based on the NHS Care Programme Approach, is regularly carried out to assess achievements within the implementation programme. A CPA group facilitate and monitor activities in this area. This concept has promoted a multidisciplinary team approach, which continues to be built on.

Seclusion

Seclusion is actively monitored by ward-based staff and regularly audited as part of the clinical audit programme. A seclusion monitoring and review group exists to monitor the findings and outline actions for improvement, where relevant. Since the introduction of audit and monitoring activities, clear and demonstrable improvements have been made, in this and other key areas of care and treatment, and have contributed to the ongoing development of teamwork.

WHERE DO WE GO FROM HERE?

Translating Theory into Practice

There has been no rigorous research or formal evaluation of multidisciplinary teamwork and treatment planning over the past 30 years, so it is difficult to measure the successes and the failures in scientific terms. Recent empirical research studies are paying serious attention to the development and importance of teamwork in health care. At Broadmoor Hospital, the past five years have seen the introduction of explicit standards and monitoring in this area. In my role as Quality Improvement Service Manager, through the monitoring of quality standards, analysis of complaints and close liaison with the hospital Patients' Council, I have seen that the changes and improvements in this area of care and many others have demonstrably improved. Multidisciplinary teams have come together and continue to develop collaborative methods of working. A structured treatment planning process has provided professionals with a framework on which to continue to develop a systematic approach to care and treatment provision.

We still have much to do in translating the theories of effective teamwork and treatment planning into practice, and there is an essential need for further research and evidence in this area, on which future practice can be based. Valid and reliable measures are available that focus on many aspects of teamwork and could be used, such as:

- Minnesota Job Satisfaction Scale (1967) – measuring intrinsic/extrinsic satisfaction
- Maslach Burnout Inventory (1986) – measuring levels of emotional exhaustion, personal accomplishment and depersonalisation in teams
- Role Conflict and Ambiguity Scales – measuring staff perceptions of their aims, objectives, roles and responsibilities within the team.

Focused Groups

Quality monitoring and clinical audit will continue to play a major role in bringing teams together, and agreeing common goals for improvement in clinical care and practice.

Other team and group activities such as risk management, critical incident debriefing, and training programmes are all developments which require teams to work closely together and provide opportunities to put an end to the interdisciplinary and inter-agency rivalries and protectionism that have dominated the professions over the years.

CONCLUSION

Multidisciplinary teams need to continually reappraise their philosophy and working practices to develop a cohesive and co-ordinated approach to the provision of services to our patient group. This focus must be underpinned by an inherent and implicit approach that values, respects and supports each member of the team, and the contribution they have to make.

This is a highly complex and contentious issue and the process of change in this area has been slow, almost insidious. There are many pressures that continue to affect teamwork and the professions, such as lack of resources, bureaucratic structures and systems, excessive paperwork, relationships within the team, the management of change which continually challenges traditional approaches, cost and other pressures from senior managers, and achieving contract and performance targets. A great many people have worked, and will continue to work, tremendously hard to develop real teamwork with which the highest standards of care, treatment and quality of life can continue to improve for our patient group. They depend on us for that.

I look forward to the next 30 years!

REFERENCE

Campbell-Heider, N. and Pollock, D. (1987). 'Barriers to physician–nurse collegiate: an anthropological perspective.' *Social Science and Medicine 25,* 5, 421–425.

CHAPTER 17

Research and Development

Charles Kaye and Alan Franey

IN THE BEGINNING

When the SHSA was created in 1989, the sixth (and last) of the guiding principles was: 'To promote research into fields related to forensic psychiatry'. This guideline, like most simple statements, was not a declaration *de novo*, a leap into the unknown. It represented, in many ways, the consolidation of what had gone before. The Special Hospitals had been a focus of research by interested individuals. The hospitals represented, as one eminent practitioner put it 'a unique laboratory!'.

In elaborating its basic guideline the Department of Health stated:

The Government are committed to the support and encouragement of the promotion of such research, and have acknowledged the important further contribution that the special hospitals can make in taking this work forward.

And that:

Forensic psychiatry is a relatively new and developing specialty. The RSU programme is not yet complete, and work on the provision of local forensic psychiatric services is still at an early stage. The services offered by this specialty need further evaluation, particularly with regard to current shortfalls in service provision, including that available at district level. There is, however, a serious lack of firm information both about current demand and the extent to which this is being met. There are also many other areas relating to the aetiology, the investigation and treatment of the problems posed by the mentally abnormal offender and the difficult to manage patient, which require further research by all of forensic psychiatry. (SHSA 1989)

A key component of research activity previously had been the Special Hospitals Research Unit (SHRU). This was founded in 1969 following an inquiry two years earlier by the House of Commons Estimates Committee into the Special Hospitals. The most lasting achievements of SHRU were the foundation of the Case Register and the fostering of university links with each Special Hospital. As one of their early reports described the Case Register:

> The main disadvantages of the hospitals' records for research purposes were that only a minimum of standardised information was available for current and discharged patients and all additional data had to be extracted from individual files. As none of the information had been collected in a systematic manner it was therefore of varying quantity, quality and reliability. The record systems themselves were event rather than patient orientated so that re-admission counted as new patients. This made it impossible to trace and link the patients' treatment experiences within the Special Hospitals which is basic to any detailed description of the population and to any evaluative studies. Finally, as the Estimates Committee noted, there was not systematic follow-up of discharged patients and very little post-discharge information was available. (SHRU 1977)

The SHRU itself was dissolved on the recommendation of the Director. As one commentator described it:

> The special hospital reports were generated and edited from the SHRU base and provided a first level publication for special hospital staff and related researchers. The most substantial work, however, was subsequently publicised in academic journals or monographs. The work of SHRU remained marginalised. This was partly because there was resistance from within the hospitals to the clinical researchers but partly too because the resources, initially quite good, were so rigidly channelled into two sources, principally the Case Register but with smaller amounts going to neurophysiology. (Taylor 1991)

The register had started in 1972 and, briefly, comprised a computerised record of the geographic, personal and offending status of all patients admitted to Special Hospitals since then – follow-up data, in terms of criminal records, hospital readmissions and records of death, was kept up to date for all patients who had left the hospitals. Since 1989 the register has been refined in quality and expanded in scope.

At the same time the hospitals' population was the subject of other important studies such as:

- 'Transfer of Special Hospital patients to NHS hospitals.' (Dell (1980)
- 'The attitudes and practices of Special Hospital consultants in relation to patients classified as psychopathically disordered.' (Dell and Robertson 1988)

Within the hospitals there was the nucleus of a research community with established, albeit modest, academic links between Broadmoor Hospital and the Institute of Psychiatry, the Merseyside Hospitals and Liverpool University, and Rampton Hospital and Sheffield University. Although doctors were prominent in this respect, a strong research interest existed in other professions within the hospitals, most notably in psychology and nursing.

In summary, there was awareness, interest and significant activity but – as with other aspects of the hospitals' existence – a notable absence of co-ordination and drive. The new Authority's job was to supply these and match them with resources.

THE TASKS

In a report published in 1996, one prominent research centre says:

> Forensic psychiatry maintains its high political profile. Prison populations in Britain are rising, the pressure on secure beds in the NHS is intolerable, individual incidents (such as the Dunblane Massacre) make headline news, and all teaching centres are now trying to develop forensic psychiatry departments. Paradoxically academic resources in forensic psychiatry are very low. (Institute of Psychiatry and the Maudsley Hospital 1996)

The SHSA faced a similar position in 1989. There was a determination to bring it positively and decisively into the research environment but first a structure had to be fashioned to sustain and foster quality research. The Authority's designated Director of Research was Dr (later Professor) Pamela Taylor. She herself was prominent in the field was an ideal leader, determined to see advances made but not prepared to take short-cuts and sacrifice thoroughness and quality. The Chief Executive had spent four years as a member of the Medical Research Council's grant-making committees and was keenly aware of the value and importance of research.

This importance was summarised in an early report to the SHSA:

The potential beneficiaries of research, they say, are therefore:

o Patients, as a result of improved understanding of their problems and of the clinical services required to deal with them

o Staff, through informed practices and professional development

o The organisation, by establishing its reputation and providing quality assurance. (Taylor 1991)

The group further underlined the functions of research in the following ways:

(a) In the context of a special hospital, research provides the basis of knowledge of the links between mental disorder and dangerous behaviour.

(b) All disciplines which claim a professional competence are ultimately dependent on research to validate the theoretical assumptions and beliefs on which their procedures and practices are based.

(c) Involvement in research facilitates professional development.

(d) Research aimed at monitoring the outcome of clinical procedures is necessary for quality assurance.

(e) Active research programmes are necessary to establish the claims of an institution to be a centre of excellence. Such a reputation attracts better qualified staff, and influences the morale of existing staff. It also influences professional bodies who approve institutions for training purposes.

What had to be assembled were the components to facilitate research. The most obvious need was financial backing – a research budget was created by the Authority under the direct control of the Director of Research. Next was the requirement for suitable researchers; there was, and still is, a shortage of fully trained health professionals who are experienced in research methods and are interested in applying their skills in the field of forensic psychiatry.

An initial step was to create a focus in each hospital by formally designating a key individual as each hospital's Director of Research. Two of the posts were filled by psychiatrists, the third by a psychologist.

Around these individuals there gathered the nucleus of a hospital research community with a formal committee and a local research newsletter. Within each hospital there was strong support, organisationally and financially, from the major disciplines.

These initial moves were reinforced by a strong focus on training posts, particularly in forensic psychiatry, with the holders being actively encouraged to carry out original research projects during their tenure.

At the same time much effort was invested in building up a formal academic presence in each hospital. A key aim was to establish a University Chair on each site. This required substantial investment by the Authority – since the universities were not in a position to contribute financially – and the creation of a suitable environment. Within the lifetime of the SHSA, two professorships were created: firstly, a Chair at Ashworth Hospital, linked to Liverpool University, which was filled by Professor Ron Blackburn, previously Head of Psychology at Park Lane Hospital and an outstanding researcher in the field of personality disorder. Secondly, a Chair at Broadmoor Hospital, linked to the Institute of Psychiatry in London, which was filled by Professor Taylor herself. A third Chair was created in 1997 at Rampton Hospital, linked to Sheffield University, building on work started under the SHSA.

These new academic departments were to be the foundation for a new generation of researchers and projects. Undoubtedly this was a major achievement giving concrete expression to the Authority's aims. In itself, however, it was not an answer, rather the establishment of a means towards the eventual goal. Much would depend on personality and leadership and the interprofessional rivalries, which do regrettably surface, could occasionally be detected. The very need to bring all professions together in a multidisciplinary context made the task harder and the goal more ambitious. But from the beginning there was a recognition of the contribution of each profession and a determination that research was not to be seen as the preserve of any one profession. As with so many other of the changes that the SHSA introduced, this was not immediately or enthusiastically greeted by all. From the headquarters projects were initiated early on that involved researchers from the Prison Medical Service, the Inner London Probation Service and nursing practitioners.

STRUCTURES

Overall direction of the research effort was maintained from the centre, at SHSA HQ. Such close interest and scrutiny was essential as the early tender shoots of investment appeared. Thus the Director of Research established regular meetings with the hospital Directors as a group and, linked to that group, other key individuals. The Director also prepared an annual report for the SHSA which both informed them about targets and progress and gave them the opportunity to raise key issues directly with Authority members.

As the SHSA developed the concept of contract-like agreements between itself and each hospital, it seemed appropriate to include a specific hospital research contract as part of that process. In this way the nascent hospital research department could express its aspirations and also accept its responsibilities for reporting on its use of resources. So too the hospitals' General Managers were drawn into the research environment since they became responsible for the hospital's commitment to the research contract. Through this chain the aim was to knit research closely into the fabric of the hospital and not have it suspended, *in vacuo*, as an optional extra.

The hospital focus, while entirely appropriate, since that reflected the working reality, did present some problems. There was the customary centrifugal tension with hospitals sometimes eager to go it alone. One interesting example of this was the question of ethical approval of proposals.

Each hospital had its own Ethics Committee and separate Research Committee. On occasion there could be conflict between these two committees when examining the same proposal. This could be exacerbated when an Authority-wide proposal needed to clear the hurdles three times. Disagreement by any one committee could halt the whole process and lead to further rounds of revision and consultation. This was a difficulty which the wider NHS has had to tackle with the creation of Multi-Centre Research Ethics Committees.

The NHS Executive were forced to create a mechanism to overcome this very problem; to quote their advice:

One Multi-centre Research Ethics Committee (MREC) will be set up in each English region. An MREC's advice will be given to LRECs in every locality involved, not just those within its host part of the United Kingdom. Once MREC approval has been obtained LRECs in every locality involved will have the opportunity to accept or reject the protocol for local reasons. The MREC will advise on research proposals which will be carried out within five or more LRECs' geographical boundaries. (NHS Executive 1997)

This circular seeks to minimise the snakes and ladders hazards which researchers proposing wide-scale projects might encounter. Within the Special Hospitals under the SHSA there was thought being given to some central ethical focus but the decision about changing the shape of service put that to one side.

Another important feature of a concerted approach to research was the organisation of conferences, on a multidisciplinary and international basis, to review progress in key areas. Thus in 1991 the Authority sponsored a two-day conference on 'psychopathic disorder'. The proceedings were later published in a special issue of the journal *Criminal Behaviour and Mental Health* (1992); as always, this linked to practical issues of treatment; as the introduction commented:

The seminar was set up to start the process of clarifying the clinical concepts underlying the legal labelling, and the full range of treatments that ought thus to be on offer. We also wanted to tackle such practical questions as whether the present tendency towards piecemeal approaches to treatment appropriately reflects the diagnostic heterogeneity, and the extent to which the legal classification embraces a group homogeneous enough to merit extension of small community (ward) concentration of intensive, psychological, specifically targeted approaches to treatment. A working group set up to maintain the momentum of these and even more fundamental challenges posed by the speakers and the invited multidisciplinary delegates from a wide range of clinical and non-clinical settings has found itself without many answers, but with a better defined set of questions and testable hypotheses about appropriate ways forward.

Such conferences, where research findings were shared, and new ideas examined, were a feature of the entire life of the SHSA with the last in 1995 focusing on psychopathic disorder (a joint conference with colleagues from the Dutch TBS) and on services for women.

PRACTICAL EXPRESSIONS

Alongside the development of the structure of research, actual projects were being pursued.

The SHSA established its commitment to research by quickly accepting responsibility for the Case Register and, subsequently, under the guidance of Professor Taylor, making substantial investment to widen its scope and relevance. This work continues today under the aegis of the Broadmoor Hospital Research Directorate.

The Authority also took over responsibility for the important benchmarking survey of Special Hospital patients (Maden *et al* 1995). Published in 1995 this work described a cross-section of patients and made a critical assessment of their need for treatment and security.

This short account is not intended to give a comprehensive overview of research in the Special Hospitals over the SHSA's lifetime, but it may be helpful to note briefly three areas of particular interest.

1. In her first research report to the Authority, Professor Taylor identified the area of 'treatment resistant' schizophrenia as one suitable for further research. This initial interest materialised into a large-scale longitudinal study involving all three special hospitals and Carstairs hospital in Scotland. This project continues currently with interesting interim reports (Taylor *et al.* in press; The Special Hospitals Treatment Resistant Schizophrenia Research Group 1996).

2. The Authority commissioned a full study of current practice with regard to the use of seclusion. This work (Mason 1993) led to the complete review and reorientation of this technique within the hospitals which itself was a significant ingredient in helping to change the hospitals' prevailing culture (as described elsewhere in this book).

3. The subject of women patients and the appropriateness of their being treated in Special Hospitals is itself contentious. One characteristic of women patients often noted is their propensity to harm themselves by self-inflicted physical abuse ('self-harm'). Research into this important area has been conducted both at Rampton and Ashworth Hospitals (Swinton and Hopkins 1996; Swinton and Smith 1997)

In addition, contributions were made to the Department of Health/Home Office review of services for MDO (Reed 1994). Dr Taylor chaired the research advisory group, many of whose recommendations have been actively pursued, not least by Dr Dilys Jones and the HSPSCB.

SHSA fellowships were created linking the Institute of Criminology with the Institute of Psychiatry and the Special Hospitals. Two holders pursued research and a further degree through these fellowships.

CONCLUSION

The SHSA cannot, and would not, claim to have 'invented' research in Special Hospitals. But its determination and investment brought research much more to the foreground in both clinical and managerial terms. Within its own short life it commissioned and carried out important studies which altered practice and through the three chairs which it helped establish it created essential focal points in each hospital.

The discipline of research contracts and annual reports created an alliance between managers and researchers that echoed the essential link between practice and research:

> Treatment is generally regarded as having two major components – the general, which includes the overall management and service strategies and the delivery of care, and the specific, which is to change or resolve presenting problems. With respect to the general, clinical research must inform service provision, both directly and through epidemiology, and in turn be applied to evaluate the provisions as they are implemented. It must inform and monitor the efficacy of specific treatments. (Taylor 1997)

The factors that led to the SHSA's emphasis and investment still remain; the requirement for quality research is as urgent as ever. The work described here has helped to provide a good basis for the future.

REFERENCES

Criminal Behaviour and Mental Health (1992) 'Psychopathic Disorder' *Criminal Behaviour and Mental Health 2*, 2

Dell, S. (1980) 'Transfer of Special Hospital patients to NHS hospitals.' *British Journal of Psychiatry 136*, 222–234.

Dell, S. and Robertson, G. (1988) 'The attitudes and practices of Special Hospital consultants in relation to patients classified as psychopathically disordered.' Maudsley Monographs No.32. Oxford: OUP.

Institute of Psychiatry and the Maudsley Hospital, Research Report 1996. London: Institute of Psychiatry.

Maden, T. *et al.* (1995) *Treatment and Security Needs of Special Hospital Patients.* London: Whurr Publishers.

Mason, T. (1993) *Seclusion Theory Reviewed, Medicine, Science and the Law 33*, 95–102.

NHS Executive (1997) *Ethics Committee Review of Multi-Centre Research – HSG(97)32.* Leeds: NHS Executive.

Reed (1994). *Review of Health and Social Services for Mentally Disordered Offenders.* London: HMSO.

SHRU (1977) *Special Hospitals Case Register – The First Five Year.* SHRU.

SHSA (1989) *Policy Guidelines.* London: Department of Health.

Swinton, M. and Hopkins, R. (1996) 'Violence and self injury.' *Journal of Forensic Psychiatry 7*, 3, 563–9.

Swinton, M. and Smith, S. (1997) 'Costs of physical health care for self injuring patients.' *Psychiatric Bulletin 21*, 9.

Taylor, P. (1997) 'Clinical Research and Forensic Psychiatry.' Delivered to the Cropwood Conference, March.

Taylor, P.J. (1991) *Research Strategy for the Special Hospitals, Feb 1991.* Unpublished report to SHSA.

Taylor, P.J., Leese, M., Williams, D., Butwell, M., Daly, R. and Larkin, E. (in press) 'Mental disorder and violence: a special hospital study.' *British Journal of Psychiatry.*

The Special Hospitals Treatment Resistant Schizophrenia Research Group (1997) 'Schizophrenia violence, clozapine and risperidone: a review.' *British Journal of Psychiatry* (suppl.31) 21–30.

PART 5

Scrutinies and the World Outside

CHAPTER 18

The Mental Health Act Commission

William Bingley

INTRODUCTION

'It is inevitable that the relationship between a service provider and the organisation charged with monitoring aspects of its work will not always run smoothly and the relationship between the Commission and the SHSA (The Authority) has been no exception' (HMSO 1995). So commented the Commission's Sixth Biennial Report, which coincided with the end of the Authority. It will be some time before an objective judgement can be made as to whether the relationship between the two organisations did, as was claimed in that report, make a genuine contribution to improving the care and treatment of Special Hospital patients.

The Commission's task is fourfold: to protect the interests of detained patients (by way of visiting detained patients in hospital, investigating complaints and monitoring the operation of the 1983 Act); to administer the consent to treatment safeguards in the Act; to review the decisions of the Special Hospital managers to withhold patients' mail; and to report on its activities every two years to the Secretary of State and Parliament by way of a Biennial Report.

From its establishment in 1983, the Commission devoted a significant amount of its resources to visiting each of the high security hospitals and, whilst the arrangements for such visits changed over the years, they continued to be accorded a high priority. With the creation of the Authority, the Commission for the first time was presented with an autonomous body with overall responsibility for the management of the three high security hospitals. In general terms, it was agreed that hospital-specific issues would be pursued with each of the hospitals, but that matters of a more strategic nature or which were of serious concern would be raised with the Authority.

THE LEGACY

When the authority came into existence on 1 July 1989 the Commission had been visiting the high security hospitals for seven years. It had been criticised 'for becoming involved in what many regarded as trivial complaints at ward level at the expense of broader and substantive issues that related to the whole Special Hospital system' (HMSO 1991).

Such criticism, which was to an extent justified, resulted in part from the limitations of the Commission's statutory remit, the principle focus of which is to visit individual detained patients, and also from the fact that prior to the creation of the Authority, there was no coherent management structure with overall responsibility for all three hospitals. At the same time, prior to 1989, the relationship between the Commission and each of the hospitals had been difficult, with each demonstrating various degrees of defensiveness. The Commission's comments in its first report that 'Commissioners were seen by many staff as yet another body whose principal task would be to find fault' and 'that the initial suspicion had not been easily or totally overcome' remained true to varying degrees throughout the 1980s. At the same time it was also true that the Commission's fear, expressed in the same report, that patients would have 'an exaggerated belief in what the Commission could do' and, by implication, when they discovered this was not true would regard it as toothless, was also justified.

An exhaustive survey of the mechanisms by which the Commission related with the high security hospitals is inappropriate and unnecessary, save to emphasise the fact that the Authority for the first time provided the Commission with an opportunity to pursue the more strategic concerns that developed out of the undertaking of its statutory responsibilities in each of the hospitals. What were they in 1989?

A review of the Commission's Biennial Reports between 1983 and 1989 reveals a number of major concerns, all of which should be seen within the context of the overriding challenge to those providing high security services: the need to find the right balance between the requirements of security and the pursuit of the therapeutic objectives which must be the ultimate justification for the existence of the hospitals. The Commission was anxious about a considerable number of matters including the following.

Patient Privacy and Conditions for Patient Care

In its First Biennial Report the Commission noted that 'physical conditions for patients and staff are poor and impede patient care'. Whilst improvements were achieved in parts of each hospital during the 1980s many areas remained grim. In 1987 the Commission expressed grave concern about overcrowding at

Broadmoor Hospital, especially in Dorset House where conditions were wholly unacceptable (HMSO 1987).

Consent to Treatment Safeguards

Implementation of the consent to treatment safeguards in the Mental Health Act, especially by doctors, was, with some shining exceptions, abysmal. Indeed, such was the Commission's exasperation, in its Second Biennial Report it specifically reported that the reluctance of one consultant at Broadmoor Hospital to use the second opinion procedure had been the subject of discussion with the Department of Health.

Patient Complaints

The absence of a patients' complaints policy and procedure common to all three high security hospitals was the subject of repeated and vigorous condemnation.

Seclusion

The use of seclusion in the hospitals and the absence of a common policy and procedure for all three hospitals was frequently raised by the Commission. Following the publication of the Mental Health Act Code of Practice in 1990, both the Authority and the Commission identified the incorporation of its guidance into such a policy as a priority.

Rehabilitation

The Commission took a keen interest in rehabilitation and especially the adequate provision of escorted leave for patients as part of the assessment of their readiness to move on. Throughout the 1980s the Commission frequently expressed its anxieties about what appeared to be the application of inadequate resources to this aspect of the hospital's work.

The Care and Treatment of Black and Ethnic Minority Patients

In its First Biennial Report (HMSO 1985), the Commission first reported to the Secretary of State and Parliament its concerns about the care and treatment of black patients under the Mental Health Act, and in its Third Biennial Report (HMSO 1989) it specifically referred to the care and treatment of such patients in the Special Hospitals and what appeared to be their clearly disproportionately high number.

Women in the Special Hospitals

The admission of, and the provision of care to, women in the Special Hospitals was another major concern of the Commission, first highlighted in its Fourth Biennial Report (HMSO 1991).

Transfer Delays

Throughout the 1980s the Commission frequently drew attention to the difficulties experienced in transferring patients from the high security hospitals to other units or the community.

THE STRATEGIC OBJECTIVES OF THE SHSA

It was against this background that the Authority and the Commission had to create a working relationship that was constructive, but not too intimate and therefore inappropriate for a service provider and the body charged with monitoring some of its activities. Before considering how that relationship developed and the difficulties attendant upon it, it may be helpful to review the objectives the Authority set for itself.

The Authority acquired from Ministers a set of strategic objectives which are referred to elsewhere. From the point of view of the Commission, the Authority at various points in its life appeared to identify the following general goals in order to pursue those objectives:

- The creation of a coherent management relationship with the three high security hospitals.
- The introduction of 24-hour care with open access for patients to their rooms and dormitories throughout the hospitals.
- The enhancement of the ability of 'middle management' (principally by way of the introduction of ward managers) to contribute to the generation of change within the hospitals and the pursuit of greater consistency in patient care and treatment.
- The introduction of a coherent and co-ordinated approach to the improvement of the quality of patient care and its monitoring.
- The establishment of an Authority-wide patient complaints policy and procedure.
- The establishment of an Authority-wide seclusion policy and procedure.
- An increased priority afforded to successfully transferring patients from the high security hospitals.

In terms of the Commission's concerns about the high security hospitals, the Authority's priorities seem to a great extent to resonate well with those of the

Commission. Neither party was under any illusion as to the extent of the task which, if it was to be achieved, would require not only major changes in culture, but in the long term perhaps a complete reconfiguration in the way high security services were provided. Many (including some members of the Commission) regarded the task as impossible.

The Authority achieved many of its objectives. For example, an Authority-wide complaints policy and procedure was introduced in April 1992 and thus the Special Hospitals for the first time had a coherent complaints procedure. In 1993 an Authority-wide seclusion policy was promulgated although its full implementation in each of the hospitals took considerably longer. The progress made in the introduction of 24-hour patient care has been a significant achievement. In its Sixth Biennial Report (HMSO 1995) the Commission listed the above, together with the increased priority given to aftercare, transfers and the introduction of Ward Managers, as the major achievements of the Authority.

THE RELATIONSHIP BETWEEN THE COMMISSION AND THE AUTHORITY

Superimposed on the mechanism by which the Commission related to each high security hospital was the new relationship with the Authority itself. In formal terms it was pursued by way of meetings every six months attended by senior members of each body and in between, these were pursued primarily through the Chief Executives. It worked at a number of different levels.

Whilst the formal meetings remained the principal focus, the Commission did informally make a significant contribution to the Authority's pursuit of a number of its objectives. It was consulted extensively about the complaints policy and procedures; it nominated a former Commissioner as a member of the Authority's working party charged with drafting the Authority-wide seclusion policy; and it contributed to the thinking which led to the establishment of the Ashworth Patients' Advocacy Service. Such informal collaboration always had to be undertaken in a manner that did not compromise or appear to compromise each organisation's pursuit of its separate statutory responsibilities or the need for a monitoring body such as the Commission to maintain a certain important distance from the organisation it monitored.

The manner in which the Commission's relationship with the Authority developed was influenced by changes in the way the Commission pursued its objectives in the rest of the NHS. With the implementation of the purchasers–providers split in the NHS, the Commission began to copy reports of its visits to NHS provider units, to NHS purchasers, many of whom incorporated them into their performance management processes. In 1995 the Commission and the Authority went one stage further and agreed to collaborate over the setting and monitoring of quality standards in the high security hospitals. Under the agreement:

- at the beginning of each Authority quality standard review year, both parties were to discuss the key quality standards to be included in the service level agreements for the forthcoming year
- the Commission was to devote part of its visiting resources to examining aspects of one or more of the Authority's quality standards which fell within the Commission's statutory remit
- a liaison cycle was to be developed, consistent with the Authority quality standard monitoring and review cycle, and both organisations would share the outcome of the monitoring.

The demise of the Authority in 1996 meant that it was only partially possible to implement the agreement, but for the Commission it did appear to represent a significant new way in which it could pursue its statutory objectives without compromising the reality and appearance of independence essential to its role.

As befits the relationship between a monitor and the monitored, the relationship was not always easy and it is not difficult to discern some of the reasons.

The establishment by the Secretary of State of the Ashworth Inquiry in 1991 under the Chairmanship of the Commission's Chairman Sir Louis Blom-Cooper QC, and with three other Commissioners as members, undoubtedly caused difficulty. Whilst the Ashworth Inquiry Report (Blom-Cooper *et al* 1992) was critical of aspects of the Commission's performance in relation to the matters it inquired into, there undoubtedly was a feeling that the inquiry team should have been independent of all those organisations with responsibilities at Ashworth. Notwithstanding the fact that a significant proportion of the matters examined by the Inquiry occurred prior to the establishment of the Authority, it was the Authority who inevitably, and quite properly, had to take management responsibility for much of what had occurred and also for the implementation of the Inquiry's recommendations. Whilst it always made clear that the members of the inquiry team had been appointed in their personal capacity, the fact that they were Commissioners did, for a time, bring a degree of tension to the relationship.

More substantive were disagreements about the legitimate business of the Commission; what could the Commission properly draw to the attention of the Authority and what could it not? The Commission has a complex statutory remit which at times is difficult to interpret. Whilst it is a monitoring body, it is not an inspectorate in the conventional sense of the word. Its principle responsibilities under the Act are visitorial and, apart from a right of access to detained patients and their records, and the power to override the decision of high security hospital managers to withhold patients' mail, it has no powers. Its focus is the implementation of the Act and, in terms of presenting its comments to the Authority, this sometimes created difficulties.

A terse reference in the Commission's Fifth Biennial Report (HMSO 1993) refers to its disappointment with the standards and compliance by many Responsible Medical Officers (RMOs) in the high security hospitals with the provisions of Part IV of the Act, concerned with consent to treatment. The difficulties the Commission had experienced since its establishment in pursuing this matter was acknowledged by the report's reference to the fact that the 'concerns of the Commission may be seen by clinicians as marginal and bureaucratic'. It went on to note that 'the Commission is responsible for ensuring that the requirements of the Mental Health Act are fully met and has anxieties about the nature of consent in closed institutions, where any perceived lack of compliance by patients can have serious consequences for them in terms of parole status and the recommendations for rehabilitation and discharge'. More pungently it noted that:

> In the Commission's experience, deficiencies in the documentation required by the Act often reflect a more serious failure to address the fundamental issues of human and civil rights about which the Act is primarily concerned. These difficulties have been discussed with the Special Hospitals Services Authority and specific incidences drawn to the attention of RMOs. The response from the hospitals has not been encouraging and this reflects badly upon the professionalism of all concerned.

In relation to one security hospital during this period, the Commission had been gravely concerned, not only about compliance with the requirements of the Mental Health Act by a number of their doctors, but also about these doctors' general competency, the performance of their duties and their working relationships with other professionals. These more general concerns were drawn to the attention of the hospital and, by way of the hospital, to the Authority. The latter's response was that the general quality of its doctors was probably without the Commission's remit, although the impact of their alleged failings upon the care and treatment of the detained patients for whom they were responsible was a matter that the Commission could draw to the attention of the hospital and the Authority.

At other times Commission representations did result in a reordering of the Authority's priorities. In 1987 the Commission drew attention to overcrowding in Broadmoor Hospital especially in Dorset House, and the fact that this had been drawn to the attention of Ministers (HMSO 1987). Some improvements resulted, principally from the Broadmoor Hospital rebuild, but in 1991 continuing unacceptable conditions in part of the hospital, especially in Dorset House, were noted in the Fourth Biennial Report (HMSO 1991). In 1993 the Commission's concerns about conditions in Dorset House (especially the third floor) were reignited by information received from both patients and staff and as a consequence of unannounced night visits by Commissioners, the seriousness of the situation was notified directly to the Secretary of State in March 1994. As a consequence, the Authority, who shared the Commission's concerns, reordered its capital and revenue funding priorities and the last patients vacated Dorset House in March 1995. Similarly, in the early 1990s the absence of effective night-call alarm systems in parts of the high security hospitals was observed by the Commission, and as a consequence of urgent representations to the Authority and the Secretary of State, they had been installed throughout the hospitals by April 1994. In both cases there was essentially no disagreement between the Authority and the Commission as to the desirability of making the changes sought – their earlier implementation was an example of how a monitoring body can contribute to a reordering of priorities.

In 1995 the Commission underwent a major restructuring, the primary objective of which was to increase the quality, quantity and contact time between members of the Commission and detained patients; to improve the way in which the Commission investigated complaints; and to improve the Commission's data collection and more general use of information. For the first time in the Commission's history, teams of Commissioners were assigned to visit the high security hospitals as their primary activity. Initially the changes, which were to have a greater impact on the rest of the NHS, were unwelcome to the Authority as they appeared to be extending the Commission's inspectorial activities at a time when increased emphasis was being placed, within the NHS, on the pursuit of quality by way of accreditation and the development of quality standards and their monitoring. There was fear that the changes might result in a loss of focus on detained patients and their liberties and entitlements. In the Commission's view this was not a significant danger as the main objective was to see more detained patients and thereby more effectively pursue the Commission's principal statutory responsibility for visiting and interviewing patients in private. Ironically, from this at times heated debate arose the collaboration between the Authority and the Commission over quality standards in the high security hospitals, which, in many ways, marked the culmination of the relationship between the two organisations.

CONCLUSION

When the life of the Authority came to an end, the Commission acknowledged its achievements, but concluded that 'a great deal remains to be done'. In its sixth biennial report the Commission concluded that 'the goal of delivering consistently high standards of care, while taking adequately into account the legitimate interests of patients, staff and the wider public, continues to prove difficult to achieve in the high security hospitals, notwithstanding the progress made in recent years and the examples of good practice that can be found in each'. In their respective spheres of responsibility, both organisations were attempting to pursue their goals in very complex institutions with a controversial past and a high and unusually negative public profile. The Commission believes that its interaction with the Authority did make an important contribution to the improvement of the care and treatment of high security hospital patients and the observation of their rights and entitlements. Whether it was important enough is for others to judge.

REFERENCES

Blom-Cooper, L. *et al.* (1992) *Report of the Committee of Inquiry into Complaints about Ashworth Hospital.* London: HMSO.

HMSO (1985) *Mental Health Act Commission. First Biennial Report 1983–1985.* London: HMSO.

HMSO (1987) *Mental Health Act Commission. Second Biennial Report 1985–1987.* London: HMSO.

HMSO (1989) *Mental Health Act Commission. Third Biennial Report 1987–1989.* London: HMSO.

HMSO (1991) *Mental Health Act Commission. Fourth Biennial Report 1989–1991.* London: HMSO.

HMSO (1993) *Mental Health Act Commission. Fifth Biennial Report 1991–1993.* London: HMSO.

HMSO (1995) *Mental Health Act Commission. Sixth Biennial Report 1993–1995.* London: HMSO.

CHAPTER 19

Inquiries and Inspections

Charles Kaye and Alan Franey

THE CONTEXT

Institutions such as the Special Hospitals must expect close and sceptical scrutiny. They exercise such a degree of control over individuals confined within their walls that by their very nature they are exempt from many conventional methods of appraisal. Furthermore they focus on patients who are very ill, frequently notorious and often dangerous. Within a national climate where confidence in the proper conduct of public service is eroded (and still slipping) and where anxiety about the effectiveness of mental health care heightens with each adverse report in the media, one can expect such scrutiny to be particularly intense.

Are the public properly safeguarded? Are the patients mollycoddled? Or conversely, maltreated? Are standards set and maintained? How is risk assessed; what degree of risk (if any) is acceptable? Are patients' rights observed, or abused? Is the budget (of well over £100 million per annum, 1996–7 figures) sufficient, extravagant, well-applied or wasted? These are some of the more obvious questions that managers, politicians and the general public want answered. It is axiomatic that internal management processes alone are not sufficient for this purpose. They are essential for control but insufficient and too biased to cover all reporting and assessment needs. Hence the need for other checks and adjudications to confirm success, examine failure and improve techniques.

These scrutinies can be usefully divided into two classes (which do in some cases overlap):

1. Inspections: the regular review by independent established bodies of very specific facets of the hospitals; a regulatory or inspectorial function which is imposed; a taking of the temperature.

2. Inquiries: the appointment of an individual or a team to review the significance of an incident, or series of incidents, usually where matters are thought to have 'gone wrong'.

Both classes share some common characteristics:

- They cause perturbation within the hospital
- They make significant demands on staff
- They work on a 'snapshot' basis (what it looks like today, this week etc.).

So:

- They cannot be comprehensive
- Their criticism is powerful, painful and (often) resented
- They are not infallible.

And:

- Their fine print is usually lost – the headlines stick.

If properly pursued both processes can, and do, help make improvements but one needs to see them as the catalysts they are. Good management and effective care are not created by such scrutinies; the encouragement and assistance they provide can however be crucial to the establishment of those desirable features.

INSPECTIONS

These reviewing bodies, of which a selection is identified, have certain significant advantages:

- Explicit expertise
- Consistency
- Set standards or protocols
- Repeat reviews
- Comparison (with other sites)
- Independence
- Sanctions or penalties

Reviewing Bodies
Mental Health Act Commission
Social Services Inspectorate
Health Service Commissioners
Health And Safety Executive
Local Fire Brigade
Environmental Health Officer
Building Inspectors
English National Board For Nursing, Midwifery And Health Visiting
Royal College Of Psychiatrists
Department Of Health
Home Office
Audit Commission
Committee For Prevention Of Torture
European Education Inspectorate

Normally their terms of reference are set nationally in reference to their function. Those inspections which are iterative and return to check and re-examine will in practice add their standards to those accepted within the hospitals' canon if only because the penalties of rejecting them are unacceptable.

The relationship between management and these bodies will vary; for a specific example of this see Chapter 18. Ideally management will welcome other drills bringing out cores for inspection. Not infrequently there is conflict between internal and external views of the significance of what has been observed. In general terms it has to be seen as part of the proving of management – these visitors offer informed opinions requiring attention and response and a hospital will lose (recognition, permission etc.) if such response is not adequate. They generally form part of the accepted rhythm but their demands should not be underestimated.

There is room to question the very processes and rationale by which such bodies arrive at their criteria. The '*Quis custodiet ipsos custodes?*' argument is relevant and a more open method of testing the inspectors' hidden reasoning would be welcome. For instance the requirements for educational approval could do with more debate; and who knows how the multinational teams of the European Committee on the Prevention of Torture manage to frame criteria that apply effectively and fairly to a special hospital in England and to jails in countries with quite different social values and systems. This is not to say it cannot be done but to ask *how* it is done and how it can be tested. Similarly the role and actions of the MHAC which is essentially focused on *individuals'* rights under the 1983 Mental Health Act; when does the concern over the situation of individuals mutate or aggregate into the justifiable criticism of the system? Is it a product of quantity or severity; how are those components balanced?

These important questions need to be put alongside the too ready acceptance of inspectorially identified blemishes. There is a Gresham's law of reported inspection where the 'bad' identified tends to obliterate the good; a properly managed review process will support the latter while helping to reform the former.

Behind the formal processes, of course, lie other scrutinies less architectural but equally influential: from the media, from pressure groups (MIND, SANE WISH, NSF), from political figures:

> MPs today demanded an urgent review of 'rehabilitation' trips by Broadmoor patients after the escape. (*Reading Evening Post* 1993)

INQUIRIES

> There *are* people to blame, and we must blame them. (Headline about the Hillsborough Inquiry in London *Evening Standard* 1996)

More arhythmic in occurrence and far more questionable in intent and effectiveness is the plethora of inquiries which regularly punctuated the SHSA's existence. In difficult circumstances, where grave events posed serious questions (and there was, and will be, no shortage of such within the high security service, however provided) a frequent response was to appoint an inquiry team. This could be done quickly; it showed concern, introduced formal scrutiny and promised considered action after an appropriate period. This technique was used to investigate escapes, absconsions,[1] murders, suicides, deaths, serious injury, hostage-taking, and allegations of ill treatments and of poor care. It was three times used to review a whole hospital (Rampton Hospital in 1989 and Ashworth Hospital in 1991/2 and, again, in 1994).

What is clear in retrospect (with infallible hindsight) is that insufficient thought or questioning went into the setting up of the galaxy of inquiries whose stars individually shone brightly but collectively often bedazzled and even blinded.

They met some needs but significantly failed in others, sometimes through inexperience, occasionally thorough bad planning, and, in instances, through

---

1 In Special Hospitals' parlance an escape is made from inside the hospital, an absconsion during a trip outside.

sheer inappropriateness. Usually the inquiry was employed as a knot to bind to-gether divergent factors operating in different planes on the false assumption that one overview could be comprehensive and fair. In this the SHSA was no different from other public bodies reacting in equivalent situations; often there was intense pressure from the Department of Health for specified action and on three occasions, all in 1991 (the Ashworth Inquiry, the first escape from Broad-moor Hospital and the Blackwood[2] Inquiry), the process was significantly led by the Department itself. The tensions between blame and learning, individual conduct and the working of systems, clinician and management, policy and op-erational reality, victims and carers, are not readily balanced. The ever-present call for speed and simplification threatens the balanced approach and the thoughtful reception of an inquiry's findings. Always present there is bias that hindsight imposes. As James Reason describes it:

> Outcome knowledge dominates our perceptions of the past, yet we remain largely unaware of its influence. For those striving to make sense of complex historical events, familiarity with how things turned out imposes a definite but unconscious structure upon the antecedent actions and conditions. Prior facts are assimilated into this scheme to make a coherent causal story... (Reason 1990)

PURPOSE OF INQUIRIES

There have been a number of formulations in this respect. Professor John Mar-tin in 1984 set out four criteria for a *successful* inquiry (Martin 1984):

- o Allaying public alarm
- o Discovering the facts and passing judgement on what took place
- o Providing an adequate explanation for what had happened
- o (In the longer term) providing a good basis for developing higher standards of care.

Sir Louis Blom-Cooper (by now the doyen of inquiry leaders) set out a slightly different quartet (referring specifically to public inquiries) (1993):

- o Establishing the facts
- o Identification of individual culpability
- o Surveying the arrangements that led to the scandal, disaster or abuse
- o Holding up to obloquy the actions that threatened public confidence.

---

2   In this chapter, where published reports include named patients, we will use those names since they are a matter of public record.

This might be termed the minatory approach. In the best investigative tradition, 'someone's got to pay for this'.

Reder and Duncan summarise the position: 'However, the more reports we read, the more it is apparent that they [inquiries] are set up to serve diverse purposes, primarily discipline, learning, catharsis and reassurance'.

Guidance from the Department of Health (HSG (94) 27 – paras 33 to 36) requires an independent inquiry in the case of homicide[3] and a local multidisciplinary audit in the case of suicide. A nice system of priorities established using public safety as the predominating criterion! This is a reality which it is easy to overlook from within the high security service. The concern for patients as individuals while recognised and supported governmentally comes second to questions of danger (actual or potential) to the public. It was not accidental that 'public protection' was set as the first term of the SHSA's mission when it was established in 1989. To this concern is directly linked the imperative succinctly if bluntly put by the headline above. For the public at large, the identification and punishment of a guilty party (or more than one) is probably the most important objective. Risk, negligence or error are not distinctions which the public wishes to see drawn. If something goes seriously wrong, someone is to blame and should be punished. Within an organisation the reaction (perhaps somewhat protective) is to seek to understand the chain of circumstances leading to an event and to learn how such a concatenation can be avoided in future. In precarious ventures, such as the rehabilitation of Special Hospital patients – where risk is inevitable and knowledge incomplete – the theme is learning to improve rather than punishing to deter. It is not negligent to make a decision which later turns out to be wrong, provided we reached that decision after assembling relevant and accessible information. All of us make errors; what is necessary is to learn from them. From within we tend to be more sympathetic to the difficulty of drawing a clear line between error and negligence and, properly, more aware of the difficulties inherent in assessing complex situations under pressure.

Inquiries should also meet the needs of victims and families to be heard, to receive explanations, to hear what action is to be taken and, if appropriate, to see blame apportioned.

However, there seems little doubt that the key motivations behind most inquiries – within and outside the Special Hospitals – is the reassurance of the public. A key component of this reassurance is blaming (individuals) and shaming (organisations). The 'simple' facts assimilated to prevent repetition by changing systems and rules is next in order of priority. Learning, the consistent

---

3   This requirement has initiated a series of inquiries which, cumulatively, has become counterproductive (see Reder and Duncan, Carson and Eastman in J. Peary (1996))

application of relevant standards and the motivation of staff, lags lamely behind.

PROCESS AND EXPERIENCE

To illustrate the SHSA's work and experience in this vexed area, it is helpful to look at linked series of inquiries at each hospital and then attempt to draw out some principles and lessons which should be helpful to present and future managers of such services. The sequences we have selected are:

Rampton Hospital

1.Prejudice and Pride, 1990

2.The Death of Bryan Marsh, 1992 – two reports

3.The Escape of Paul Marshall, 1994

Broadmoor Hospital

The deaths of

1.Michael Martin, 1984

2.Joseph Watts, 1988/9

3.Orville Blackwood, 1991/3

Ashworth Hospital

1.The Ashworth Inquiry, 1991/2

2.Investigation into Alternative Literature, 1993

3.With Care in Mind Secure (Hospital Advisory Service 1995)

Within each sequence we will briefly set out relevant events, describe key processes and identify outcomes, both positive and negative. Analysis, of course, will not identify the individuals concerned and it should be understood that detailed comments about the situation at particular hospitals are historical commentary to illustrate process.

THE VALUE OF CRISIS: RAMPTON HOSPITAL

1. Prejudice and Pride

In October 1989, a team of four very experienced and senior health service professionals were commissioned by the Department of Health and the SHSA:

> To report upon the present state of Rampton Hospital ten years after Sir
> John Boynton's Review, to look into the hospital from the outside and to
> look outwards from the hospital; to look at the total use of resources, both in

producing the best possible distribution of services and the effect on clinical outcomes, including the influence of security; whether the hospital is concentrating on services which only a special hospital could and should offer; to consider future possibilities for the whole range of services provided by the special hospital services. (SHSA 1989)

In many ways it was a HAS (Health Advisory Service) review of the whole hospital. It was not accidental that the team included a former director of the HAS. The team spent ten working days in the hospital, visited 'almost all wards and departments at least once' and interviewed patients, staff and other interested parties. It produced a thoughtful and detailed report (Dick *et al.* 1990) which earnestly sought to meet all of its terms of reference. It was not uncritical in its assessment:

We visitors approached the task of reviewing the progress of the hospital since Sir John Boynton's report of ten years ago, with prejudice like anyone else. Our expectations were low and we could not entirely believe that all which was claimed in the briefing material supplied to us about the hospital, could be trusted. (p.4)

But overall their conclusion was positive:

What we found was a hospital in good health and capable of solving problems. We talked to a lot of people, both on their own and in groups and went to each ward and department, usually unannounced and informally as mentioned in the description of our method of working.

We are able to conclude that Rampton Hospital has put the past of ten years ago behind and now has pride in what it is doing. We did not meet complacency. There are still many problems and plenty to do but there is much at the hospital which compares favourably with many NHS psychiatric hospitals. (p.4)

The report then reviews briefly most of the key areas within the hospital and speculates quite widely about the future of Rampton Hospital and indeed the Special Hospital Service concluding:

for these reasons, the 'territorial model' which integrates local and special services, and which can absorb evolutionary changes in health care delivery, is the best choice (p.46)

At the beginning of the SHSA's life the tenor of this document was immensely reassuring. It indicated that the hospital had moved on from the Boynton Report ten years before and now apparently presented a quite different picture. Not everything was perfect but the indications all round were encouraging.

In retrospect this confidence was in part misplaced. Clearly there was good work being carried out and many bad practices had been expunged but subsequent events suggested that this initial *tour d'horizon* had missed some significant features which were perhaps entrenched rather than prominent.

2. The Death of Bryan Marsh

On 31 May 1992 a 42-year-old patient, Bryan Marsh, who had been resident in the hospital for 12 years, solitary, overweight, a heavy smoker, died following an incident on Elms Ward.

The 'incident' appears to have followed this course; Mr Marsh verbally abused a female nurse which led the Charge Nurse to approach him. A physical altercation followed, control and restraint techniques were applied to the patient who was put in seclusion where he collapsed and died. The whole episode lasted about 40 minutes.

The police were called in and the internal hospital inquiry decided to focus on 'Organisational, Operational and Managerial issues'. Given police interest the 'immediate circumstances' were not to be addressed. The report of this first inquiry commented on issues such as arrangements for dealing with emergencies, staff training and post-incident support to staff. It did not consider why Mr Marsh had died. However the police action, in questioning staff 'under caution', made clear that the report the hospital had completed did not deal with the heart of the incident – the death and the cause.

The SHSA decided to set up its own inquiry team headed by the Director of Security. That report was completed by September 1992 and presented a very critical assessment. It felt the whole incident on the ward was badly handled, that staff were evasive in giving evidence, that training for, and use of, Control and Restraint techniques were deficient and that senior managers had mishandled the aftermath of the incident. Notable in this report was the importance attached to the evidence of other patients. This evidence conflicted with that given by the staff. Following this report the Charge Nurse was dismissed for gross misconduct. The coroner's court in 1994 recorded an open verdict; this followed an unsuccessful attempt to prosecute members of the ward staff for conspiracy and manslaughter.

Behind this bold recital of facts lie several key realities. The hospital management regarded the death as an almost inevitable part of the hospital's work; thus their review side-stepped the key question of 'why' and 'how' electing to leave that to the police (a necessarily slow process with no certainty about the outcome). The hospital deeply resented the role of the SHSA in forcing upon it a second inquiry which revealed major shortcomings in attitudes and actions.

From the centre in London it was difficult to judge which should be more worrying: that staff had behaved unprofessionally and tried to cover up what they had done; or that local management had failed almost entirely to see the significance of this patient's death and considered the centre's concerns to be misplaced and hostile.

All this was a far cry from 'a hospital in good health'. The familiar defensiveness of the closed institution was strongly in evidence and learning was to be confined to technicalities (of resuscitation and first aid) which were insignificant compared to the very real deficits in staff, nurses and managers, revealed by further investigation.

3. The Escape of Paul Marshall

In 1994 a patient on Hawthorns Villa completed his preparations for a successful escape. He left the traditional pillow in place in his bed to camouflage his absence, slipped out of the ward's back door and over a weak spot in the perimeter wall which he had previously reconnoitred.

Any escape from within the hospital's perimeter represents a major failure on the part of the service and cannot be excused. As might be expected (and quite properly) this lapse attracted national media coverage and a full investigation was held. Much of the obvious emphasis was on improving the physical security and the report prompted a major investment in strengthening the protective barrier around the hospital.

More significant however were the findings about the ward regime and their hospital-wide implications. Firstly the laxity of the ward's organisation had allowed preparations for the escape to be completed and then allowed a whole night to lapse before the patient's absence was noted. That was bad enough and staff were disciplined. More fundamental however was the revelation that the ward team – the mutual co-operation and interdependence of trained staff – was a chimera; management thought it existed but staff knew it did not. Central to this confusion was the fact that individual consultants had their patients in many locations across the hospital making it impossible on a practical basis for the consultant to lead the ward team. The ward might have as many as seven consultants and a consultant have as many as ten wards: real leadership and consistent organisation were virtually impossible given such a spread of responsibility. Another reform required! And only implemented following strong pressure from the centre.

Behind this lay another important question, concerning the selection of patients in terms of degrees of security required: decisions had been made in isolation and clinical teams left without guidance.

These outcomes suggested very basic defects in clinical organisation which had allowed the escape to take place. The inquiry traced the dramatic event back to the root causes and the gap in the wall was not nearly as devastating as those gaps in the clinical teams which had allowed the former to be exploited.

Summary: Rampton Hospital

Complex organisations deserve subtle and thoughtful consideration. A swift broad-ranging review may produce a few helpful pointers but is unlikely to be of significant value. It might even be seen as unhelpful since a positive report could encourage complacency – as was probably the effect at Rampton Hospital in 1990. The reality is that change is gradual and piecemeal in its progress. 'Quick fixes' in terms of reviews or actions are of little value since they will not penetrate below the institutional epidermis to any layer of substance. Of course the need for reassurance often predominates; that need may be local or national and cannot be ignored, but effectiveness in reporting and assessing will start with clear and realistic objectives.

Always in institutions, or bureaucratic frameworks, there is a balance to be found between awareness and acceptance, between empathy and erosion. The initial local review into Mr Marsh's death took too much for granted; it failed to question in a disturbing way. The death – a shocking outcome – was taken as a datum, an encapsulated event, which was not to be examined. Thus questionable practices and behaviour could pass unobserved until a more detached and paradoxically more incisive approach cut through to the centre of the episode. The everyday currency of behaviour within the special hospitals is inflationary in terms of violence, threats and danger. That can blunt the sensibilities and make the extraordinary commonplace. There is a need to keep in touch with the values outside, the need to remain 'shockable': death and injury must not seem ordinary. Thus we felt it appropriate to produce at the end of 1992 'Guidance on Action Following the Death of a Patient' which opened: 'The death of any patient from whatever cause, should be regarded as an event requiring full and speedy investigation. This guidance covers deaths, both unexpected and anticipated and defines action required in both situations.' (SHSA 1992)

Thus the second lesson: that any review team drawn from inside the hospital needs to question the assumptions and not accept things readily simply because they are familiar. A combination of 'insiders' and 'outsiders' is often helpful: those who know the intrinsic difficulties of care within the institution balanced by those who will challenge freely.

Establishing the facts is only the beginning; analysing the relationships between the facts, finding the causes, is far more taxing and valuable. What started as a review of security – an obvious response to an escape – became a critique of clinical practice, requiring fundamental changes in the pattern of doctors' work. Again an 'outside' approach makes such questioning easier and is likely to expose and preserve awkward issues. In the time of the SHSA, 'outside' could and did often include senior staff from headquarters or even non-executive members who were committed to the service but not looking for sensational conclusions.

LENGTHY LEARNING: BROADMOOR HOSPITAL

Three deaths of black male patients in apparently similar circumstances prompted a series of inquiries and a learning process still being pursued.

1. Michael Martin

In 1984 Michael Martin, aged 23, was restrained by nursing staff following an incident with another patient. He was put into seclusion, stripped and injected while being restrained with sedatives. An hour and a quarter later he was found dead in the seclusion room.

The inquiry was carried out by a QC and reported in April 1985 (The Ritchie Report). It judged that his care was 'not affected by the fact of his race', that 'staff...displayed no racial prejudice' (p.38). 'No excessive force was used...but the use of a neck hold was dangerous and should not have happened'. It was because staff had not been given proper practical instructions. The patient should not have been moved from one ward to another while disturbed and the crucial injections were given without full regard to the circumstances. Finally observation after injection was inadequate.

2. Joseph Watts

Four years later, Joseph Watts died in the hospital. He was 30 years old, born in Jamaica, described as a 'gentle giant' and had been admitted in 1984. In the evening of 23 August 1988 he was involved in an incident with another patient in a ward dormitory. Both patients were removed and placed in seclusion. A nursing team – with shields and helmets – entered Mr Watt's seclusion room (the teams numbered between five and ten nurses according to different accounts). A mêlée ensued and Mr Watts, under restraint, was given an injection. Within minutes he was dead.

The inquiry team was drawn from other Special Hospitals with one additional member from the general NHS. They made recommendations about the use of Control and Restraint and training in its techniques. They were critical about the absence of any definitive seclusion policy and the failure to consider alternatives to seclusion. They were particularly concerned about staff attitudes:

> The attitudes of ward staff towards patients and their treatment and management did not, we feel, reflect the aspiration and expressed expectations of senior management within the Hospital. We heard patients referred to by ward staff in ways suggestive of patronism and infantilisation. (SHSA 1990, p.22)

And they felt:

it was depressingly clear to us that a wide gulf exists in general between 'management' and staff at ward level. (p.22)

They were also critical of several other aspects of the hospital: 'quality of life' for patients, absence of treatment plans. They recommended the use of 'outside agencies' to promote change. They referred briefly to 'racism' saying they had 'detected no sign of institutional racism' (p.25) in his treatment.

3. Orville Blackwood

Mr Blackwood died in Broadmoor Hospital in August 1991. He was then 31 years old. He was born in Jamaica and had a long psychiatric history, being admitted to Broadmoor Hospital in 1987. On the day of his death he appeared disturbed and argumentative and was asked to go into a seclusion room which he did. He stayed in seclusion refusing medication and it was decided to administer medication; a doctor and nurse entered the seclusion room to do this. He was restrained, injections given and then left in the room. He collapsed almost immediately and died.

Public reaction saw common factors between the three deaths:

- young black men
- involved in a struggle with nurses while being restrained
- secluded
- injected while under restraint
- suddenly dying.

The ethnicity of all three patients was linked to the relatively high representation of black people among the hospital's patients (between 17 and 18 per cent, similar to the proportion in the jails). This in its turn was linked to strongly held views among the black community that the Special Hospitals were being used as part of the establishment's armoury against young black males.

The SHSA wanted to know what common factors there were between the three deaths and what part, if any, racial prejudice had played. The inquiry team and its remit reflected this: independent chairman, a nurse from the Department of Health, a black academic with an established interest in mental health and a doctor from another Special Hospital, with a remit to look at all three deaths and recommend 'future policies and actions'. The report itself (SHSA 1993) was not published until the summer of 1993, being delayed until the outcome of a second inquest was known.

The report was thorough and critical. It reviewed key areas including medication, seclusion, control and restraint and race and culture. It also added an interesting rider:

Because of the deep-seated defensive (but to a degree understandable) reactions that arise in response to the type of criticisms we are making, we are concerned that our recommendations may not be implemented unless some external stimulus exists to ensure that this takes place. One remedy would be for this Inquiry Team to be invited by the Authority to reconvene in not longer than twelve months to two years to monitor and report upon the degree to which our recommendations have been implemented. (p.77)

Although the SHSA published a detailed response to all the recommendations, this particular suggestion was not accepted.

Summary: Broadmoor Hospital

This triplet of reports carried with it the increasing concerns that basic problems within the hospital were not being reviewed. Concerns voiced in the report on Michael Martin's death, (for instance, use of seclusion, use of Control and Restraint techniques, operation of the intensive care unit) were still being repeated by the report on Orville Blackwood nearly ten years later.

As that latter report expressed it:

Such a picture was painted of Broadmoor Hospital by the Inquiry into the death of Joseph Watts in 1988. The report noted 'a marked disparity between the commendable beliefs and aspirations of senior staff concerning Hospital attitudes to patients and the attitudes expressed and indicated by nursing staff at ward level'. The report described a 'gulf' between management, at all levels, and staff at ward level. It went on to strongly recommend that as a matter of top priority the Hospital Management Team seek the advice of 'outside agencies' experienced in the management of change in large institutions. The task of changing staff attitudes was described as 'challenging and urgent'.

However, in their response to the recommendation, the Hospital Management Team revealed a somewhat blasé attitude:

It is accepted that there is an additional problem with some staff but the Hospital Management Team have a clear strategy to address the management of change and, where appropriate, will consult with outside agencies. Now that the Inquiry report can be made available to the Prison Officers' Association and the Royal College of Nursing, the concerns about staff attitudes raised in the Report can be properly addressed.

It is quite clear to us that the concerns raised in the Watts Report have not been properly addressed. There remains a serious gulf between the official policies and beliefs of the Hospital Management Team and actual practice at ward level. (p.71)

Similar incidents, prompting congruent recommendations. Yet the very repetition, the patient's death, that occasioned the reports led the last team to feel that basic flaws had not been put right. They felt this to the extent that they had no confidence in management to carry out the necessary changes, to move beyond the description of new policies into their enactment. The struggle to change life on the ward remained as difficult as ever with each successive report illustrating that difficulty. Certainly the last of these reports, with the wider remit, and thorough, painstaking review of key issues, provided local management with an action plan which is still being pursued, in, for example, the division of intensive care wards into smaller units, completed early in 1997; and the first comprehensive transcultural awareness course mounted in Autumn 1997.

HARSH SPOTLIGHT: ASHWORTH HOSPITAL

1. The Ashworth Inquiry

This inquiry was the most monumental, extensive and expensive of all held during the SHSA's tenure. It was appointed in April 1991, later converted into a full statutory inquiry[4], and reported in July 1992. It produced a two-volume report, running to over 500 pages, which was vigorously critical of Ashworth Hospital and indeed the Special Hospital Service.

> Indeed, we would even question the need for the Special Hospitals within contemporary forensic psychiatric services. (Sir Louis Blom-Cooper's letter to Secretary of State, 6 July 1992)

It was convened to review allegations of ill treatment of patients contained in a TV programme broadcast on 4 March 1991. Interestingly the composition of the panel was made up entirely of members of the Mental Health Act Commission including the Chairman and Vice-Chairman. This was a proposal opposed by the SHSA who felt that such individuals, by their very involvement in the Commission's work, would carry to the inquiry opinions, and perhaps prejudices, already formed.

The essence of this large-scale inquiry was not largely different from the conclusions of the Blackwood report which we have already considered.

> We are, however, aware that much good work is being done in Ashworth in developing standards and in producing an effective quality assurance programme. Many fine words were placed before us, demonstrating the commitment and enthusiasm of management to introduce these ideas. The lengthy address by Mr Charles Kaye, Chief Executive of the SHSA, on 30 March 1992 was a *tour de force* in terms of the vision of a Special Hospital

---

4   Giving it the status of a court with power to subpoena witnesses and take evidence under oath.

system that exuded excellence. His aspirations could only be whole-heartedly endorsed. But, as our expert observers often repeated, the core problem for nurses at Ashworth has been the total lack of effective nursing leadership. Without leadership there will be no change in culture, no change in the value ascribed to patients. Paper exercises will remain just so much waste paper. It is the translation of authoritative policies into high standards of care at the coalface that is desperately needed. (p.153)

The inquiry accelerated many changes already being advocated by the SHSA. It prompted the creation of a task-force to reshape the two reluctant partners in the Ashworth marriage (Park Lane and Moss Side Hospitals) into one clinical entity. Ironically, that reshaping created the specialist unit for personality disordered patients which is now itself the subject of the second public inquiry focused on the hospital.

But a public inquiry of such scope fully reported on by all the media also makes harsh demands on individuals who appear in the spotlight and on the very institution which it examines: 'Any institution which is put under the searchlight of a public Inquiry is bound to suffer in a variety of ways' (p.7).

The continuing obloquy that attached to the institution is virtually ineradicable, no matter how extensive the subsequent change. The inquiry and the negative conclusions (since such inquiries seem inevitably to draw sadly critical pictures) remains the key point of referral to which attention returns; the albatross never disappears. Indeed one might speculate on whether the second public inquiry might have been made more likely by the precedent of the first (with both set up by the same political figure).

Undoubtedly the force of the Inquiry Report contributed to the decision to review the future of the Special Hospital Service propelling it into the purchaser/provider convention by dissolving the SHSA. One expects that the operation of the service within this new context will itself be under critical scrutiny in 1997 and 1998 as the second Ashworth Inquiry reports.

2. Offensive Behaviour

One spin-off from the inquiry was the decision by the SHSA to appoint a specialist team to investigate 'offensive and racist interaction' within the hospital. The team, made up of a retired Deputy Chief Constable assisted by two other retired policemen, obviously used police investigatory methods to pursue its task. They reported that (Ord 1993):

The intimidation took four forms: personal confrontation, which was not common and rarely led to personal injury; damage to property but for which often the tangible evidence was not preserved; telephone calls for which there was never any evidence other than the victim's word; and mail, some of which had been retained but most of which had been destroyed. Some people had suffered spasmodically; some had suffered when feelings were running high at the time of industrial disputes; and some had been the victims of a sustained and prolonged campaign. The resilience and fortitude of the latter category was impressive. (p.9)

They observed staff's reaction:

Ashworth Hospital has been subjected to intense media attention. The Report had been heavily critical. The staff were under considerable pressure and reactions varied. There were those who welcomed the attention and recommendations for change: others resented the criticism and were opposed to much of what was being suggested. There were some who recognised the need for change but were sceptical about it being achieved. (p.18)

Their work led to disciplinary charges being brought against a number of staff (mostly nurses), several of whom were dismissed.

Their comment on the future with regard to management was clear:

Senior management have become heavily committed in meetings of various sorts, policy, review and reorganisation; they need to keep abreast of paper work and administrative chores. However there is a danger of being over committed to the point of entrapment. Operational supervision is a most important activity at any time but most especially at present. Visiting wards and other areas of clinical, medical and rehabilitating activity provides the opportunity to see whether professional cultural changes are real; whether attitudes have really changed; whether organisational changes are effective and whether key staff are as good as the reports on them. It also provides the opportunity to listen and to be heard at first hand. (p.20)

3. With Care in Mind Secure

As a deliberate follow-up to the Inquiry Report, the Health Advisory Service were asked to carry out a full review of the hospital's service. This they did in November 1994 and published their report in January 1995. In general they were cautiously optimistic as they scanned across the scene in the whole of the hospital:

The HAS recognises that the patients managed in the Special Hospitals Service are distinguished from those managed elsewhere in the health service by having mental disorders which require their assessment and/or management in circumstances of high security. Many have committed serious offences. Maintaining open, empathic and helping yet objective relationships with people whose acts may be or have been abhorrent requires a great deal of maturity and balance from the staff if the offences are not to be dissociated from the individuals and denied or patients avoided or mismanaged. Individual members of staff can find themselves under immense emotional strain in endeavouring to maintain helping relation- ships while holding onto awareness of patients' behaviours, past and present. Therefore, close clinical supervision and personal support are essential for the staff at Ashworth Hospital.

The HAS recognises that Ashworth Hospital and its staff have undergone major changes in the past three years. These have been guided by the SHSA and a specially commissioned Task Force and, more recently, by the SHSA and a general manager recruited to take on the challenges at Ashworth Hospital. The result has been that fundamental principles of the hospital organisation have been challenged and overhauled. The new style of the hospital that has been built upon this foundation is seen by many staff and patients to be more appropriate to the provision of the quality of services all involved would wish to see. Considerable advances have been made in providing a more rational organisational base for the delivery of patient care and, overall, a great deal of progress has been made in addressing some of the unhelpful aspects of the previous hospital culture.

The review team found that there are, however, some tensions that have either been created or have not been resolved in the process and the translation of exacting principles of care into practice has not been problem free. (NHS HAS 1995, p.2)

But they sounded some important warning notes:

Although the quality of nursing practice was often of a high order, many nurses had difficulty in identifying the skills that they were employing and in articulating their philosophy of care.

The review team considered that many nursing staff had difficulty in conceptualising the principles of care which would form the basis of a comprehensive care plan. While it was encouraging to see the attempts that were being made in respect of systematic care planning, there is considerable room for development. (p.33)

and:

CONCLUDING COMMENTS

In commenting upon the many changes which have been made at Ashworth Hospital in the last three years, the review team has acknowledged that these have, for the most part, been led from the top down.

There are a number of significant challenges still facing the staff of Ashworth Hospital. If these challenges are to be successfully met then the review team considers that it is of paramount importance that the staff of Ashworth Hospital, at all levels, work together to see the successful implementation of the development already begun. They will require a positive approach to the agenda that is facing them all. The review team considers that is of signal importance that this change agenda is not seen as a responsibility for managers and other key staff alone. Rather, success is the responsibility of all staff. All can contribute to ensuring that the changes and development wrought are to the benefit of all patients. (p.107)

Summary: Ashworth Hospital

A devastating report composed with the maximum of publicity by a team imposed upon the organisation had been followed by internal review. That review included a specially chosen task-force led by an SHSA non-executive member and a team investigating 'dirty tricks'.

Major changes in the hospital's organisation and arrangements were introduced and an impartial review two years later by an impressive multidisciplinary team (invited in by the SHSA) recorded that good progress was being made although significant work was still outstanding. It seemed that, as the Ashworth Inquiry put it: 'Only after the wound is cleansed can healing begin' (p.7).

INQUIRIES: ASSESSMENT AND CONCLUSIONS

> What I think these Inquiries are addressing is the contrast between what we can predict and what we should have known; failures and missed opportunities and what is and what might be. (Bingley 1995)

The preceding pages have sketched, in brief outline, nine inquiries that took place under the SHSA. This is far from being a complete list: these have been selected to demonstrate different approaches to inquiry-making and to give some impression of their cumulative force in each hospital, and indeed within the Authority.

Any inquiry is likely to be motivated by one or more of the following concerns:

1.   The seriousness of the event (such as death, escape)

2.   The volume of publicity

3.   The need to describe the facts

4.   The desire to learn and improve

5.   The urge to blame

6.   The need to demonstrate action and concern.

We can see the tension between the defensive and the learning: each has its own validity and neither can be ignored.

Within the inquiries we have reviewed we see paradoxically progress and repetition. Initially problem areas are identified; plans and policies are then formulated; and the process of implementation and reinforcement follows. Our broad survey suggests considerable movement in the first two phases but patchy results on the third. Good practice is more difficult to sustain than good preaching.

Some important observations from our experience:

Setting up an Inquiry

- Be aware of 'Inquiry Fatigue'; a plethora of inquiries will be self-defeating.

- Define carefully the scope of the inquiry: make it as precise as possible and make clear the limits. What does management want to learn more about?

- Consider the level at which to pitch the event – how much to rely on local personnel? What need is there for independent scrutiny?

- Select chairman and members for personal qualities first and professional background second. Ensure they accept the precise scope of the inquiry *before* appointment.

- Agree with team questions of: public or private hearings, representation of witnesses, publication of report, timetable.

- Recognise that disciplinary and/or police proceedings are separate entities and can (often must) run in parallel.

- Do not delay one form of action, waiting upon the outcome of another, that way lies paralysis and ineffectiveness (the SHSA did this with one report in the early days, waiting a year before actioning it fully – much of the impact was lost).

Using an Inquiry

- Agree how a report is to be responded to: accept in full, dispute, publish response?

- Agree procedures for following up progress with recommendations – this needs to be on two levels: initially as 'special' tasks separately pursued; subsequently integrated into organisation's tasks and objectives (but not lost sight of).

- Ensure that wisdom accumulates. Devise a system that gathers together the essence of successive reports, that uses them as a sequence of snapshots and applies what is to be revealed to the organisation. This sounds obvious but is a difficult and sophisticated task – one which needs to be carried out at several levels (a failure to do this at a national level is very noticeable; or would such an exercise be too politically embarrassing?).

o Separate learning from blame: the latter is short-term action while the former is the long-term, more important, investment. Don't confuse the two, or allow blame to become a full stop.

With hindsight we should have initiated fewer inquiries but followed them up more vigorously.

REFERENCES

Bingley, W. *Hospital Inquiries – Criminal Behaviour and Mental Health.* (1995 supplement).

Blom-Cooper, L. (1993) *Current Legal Problems 46 Part 2.* London: OUP.

Blom-Cooper, L. *et al.* (1992) *Report of the Committee of Inquiry into Complaints about Ashworth Hospital.* London: HMSO.

Evening Standard (1996) 28 November.

Dick, D. *et al.* (1990) *Prejudice and Pride.* London:

Martin, J. (1984) *Hospitals in Trouble.* Oxford: Basil Blackwell.

NHS Health Advisory Service (1995) *With Care in Mind.* Sutton: NHS HAS.

Ord, J.B. (1993) *Investigation at Ashworth Hospital.* London: SHSA.

Reading Evening Post (1993) 16 December.

Reason, J. (1990) *Human Error.* Cambridge: Cambridge University Press.

Reder, P. and Duncan, S. (1996) 'Inquiries After Homicide'. In J. Peary (ed) *Inquiries after Homicide.*

Report concerning the death of Michael Martin (The Ritchie Report) (1985).

SHSA (1989) *Prejudice and Pride.* London: SHSA.

SHSA (1990) *Inquiry into the Death of Joseph Watts.* London: SHSA.

SHSA (1992) *Guidance on Action Following the Death of a Patient.* London: SHSA.

SHSA (1993) *Big, Black and Dangerous?* London: SHSA.

CHAPTER 20

Press and Public Relations

Charles Kaye

THE ISSUES

Contemporary society, particularly as represented by the various media, wants more information and less secrecy. Contemporary institutions acknowledge the need to explain and to justify and thus to court the media. This gavotte draws the parties together to share news and aspirations; as the dance proceeds, conflict arises and the partners are soon out of step.

'Openness' means quite different things to the cameraman and to the manager. To the reporter reticence is virtually concealment and that suggests guilty secrets, lurking scandal. To the manager and the clinician, too much detail means a betrayal of trust and, often, an adverse effect on an individual, staff or patient.

While both parties want to be closer – with press conferences organised, interviews arranged, cameras 'inside' – that closeness can sometimes help, by demystifying and demonstrating, and sometimes hinder, by sensationalising. And thus the scene becomes a contest. The need to inform and to respond to the media must not, cannot, be denied but the risks attendant upon working closely with camera and reporter are equally real. 'Openness' must not be synonymous with naïveté since there cannot be boundaries round the media's involvement. The sensational is never likely to disappear – it's endemic to English media life and the Special Hospitals are only one profitable seam – but the effort to inform soberly and without damage will continue simply because it reflects a pride in the work being carried out. Our experience was mixed; we devoted much effort to an important area and learnt some painful lessons.

SETTING THE SCENE

The ambivalence that sits at the very centre of the Special Hospitals' existence is nowhere more starkly depicted than in our relationships with the media. Today's 'holiday camp' is effortlessly transformed into tomorrow's 'reign of terror'; 'brutalised patients' can also double as 'crazed murderers'. It's worth considering the nature of this ambivalence to understand better the demands of working with the media and the conflicts which frequently result from these contacts.

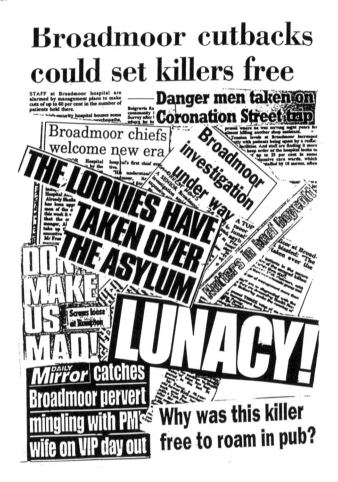

Figure 20.1 Montage of headlines

In creating high security hospitals society acknowledges a need to distinguish between individuals who are dangerous through mental illness and those whose anti-social behaviour is part of their character (and are thus placed in prison). It has designated environments (the Special Hospitals), which uniquely have two prime purposes: to detain (as a prison) and to treat (as a hospital). We have well-developed views and awareness with regard to both functions. As a society we know what detention means – it's punishment for bad behaviour;

deprivation of liberty and choice; and an uncongenial (not to say harsh) environment. Equally, we know what treatment is: care, support, therapy, opportunity for recovery, rehabilitation and a return to the community ('discharge'). Thus arises the public confusion in assessing a special hospital since the two sets of criteria (usually quite adequate and reliable) don't blend well.

This confusion reaches deeper, of course. The very distinction on which the hospitals depend – the identification of illness as a cause of behaviour – can easily be repudiated when that behaviour is so egregious as to remove all vestiges of sympathy for the patient. This is closely allied to the widespread fear (compounded by ignorance) of mental illness which dominates the public's reaction to all mental health care.

The hospitals are thus isolated social institutions whose existence uneasily acknowledges a phenomenon – violence through illness – which frightens society. Patients sent to the hospitals are made outcasts, deprived of status and rights but still the objects of intense curiosity rather like the lion in the cage, providing the same *frisson* of fear.

Indeed, that ambiguity can be seen in the hospitals themselves, which are, after all, part of this wider society. At Rampton Hospital in 1995 there was a proposal to establish a visitors centre on the outskirts of the main hospital. This was to provide accommodation, during the day and overnight, for patients' visitors and relatives who have often to undertake long and expensive journeys to get to the hospital. The centre was to back onto part of the hospital estate where staff and their families lived. The objections from those residents were vociferous, articulating the same 'nimby'[1] arguments as you would encounter anywhere in the country – but put by some of the very carers themselves!

Their role makes the Special Hospitals magnetically newsworthy, attracting virtually daily attention. Prurience and scandal are the keynotes of this focus. As a Health Authority we said from the beginning that it was part of our duty to explain our purpose and our methods and to encourage contact with the media to help that process of explanation.

In practical terms, we pursued this task in three forms: firstly by establishing the groundrules; secondly by opening communications; and thirdly by reacting vigorously to distorted and prejudicial reports.

THE GROUNDRULES

We knew that we must try to accommodate and harmonise conflicting interests. If we wanted better reporting, we had to offer press and TV opportunities to learn about our work, meet our staff and patients and question what we were

---

1 'Not in my backyard'.

doing. But in that process there were – and are – significant risks. Risks to our institutions and service, certainly, in terms of distortion and poor reporting but, more importantly, risks to staff and patients.

The media need the testimony of the individual to convey the message. Make an individual's vulnerability incandescent and, they say, you can best and most graphically illustrate your point. If by the intensity of that scrutiny you cause further damage, if by simplifying issues in the personalising you lose the broader theme, it is still a good story.

Essentially the media's relationship with individuals is transitory – a brief spotlight; the Special Hospital relationship is long-term and has to include dealing with the unforeseen consequences of passing stardom. An individual may be nationally identified and branded by a two-minute interview on a national channel. So, the presence of cameras may tempt a patient into the spotlight without his giving thought to the longer-term consequences when anonymity is important to his re-entry into society. Similarly the reporting of a 'scandal' story can damn members of staff nationally and irrevocably before any process of evaluation is completed and any balanced judgement made.

We decided that we must produce guidelines which would meet the different interests and give all involved – media, patients and staff – some principles

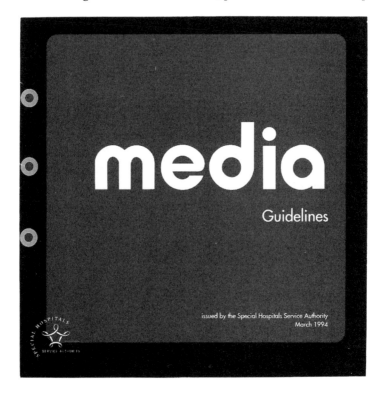

Figure 20.2 SHSA media guidelines

to rely on. These guidelines, drafted after a long consultation, were published early in 1994. We deliberately produced them in an eye-catching format to emphasise their relevance and topicality:

The twin themes of the contents (the text is given in Appendix 3) were rights and responsibilities centred around the primary duty of confidentiality. We dealt with difficult issues such as patients wishing to contact the media, the relationship between staff and their patients in the face of media attention, written contracts with the media and the role of the clinical team.

The existence of these guidelines and the presence of an experienced public relations manager in each hospital enabled us to be more purposeful in this area. They didn't solve all the problems but they did provide an essential and consistent frame of reference.

OPENING COMMUNICATIONS

It's important to stress that this was not an 'open doors' policy. The very nature of the hospitals' work means that access will always be restricted and controlled. However, there was – and is – scope for reporting of events, sharing of plans, identification of success and, importantly, explanations when things go wrong. A key component in such a strategy is to have a competent and well-informed spokesman available: not a 'spin doctor' to gloss over the unpalatable but an individual with the authority and conviction to be honest. Even this apparently self-evident common sense approach aroused anxieties. Government departments are ultra-sensitive about releasing stories which might have the potential for political embarrassment, or which could be used as ammunition within other contexts. Our view of good media relations was not always theirs – or that of their press office. The tensions were not solely between hospitals and media.

In this more open climate, there is a central distinction to be made between the local and the national media with the former much more disposed to presenting the positive as well as the negative. Nationally, as far as the special hospitals seem to be concerned, good news is usually no news. Furthermore, it's quite clear that Broadmoor Hospital has a far higher media profile than its two sister hospitals. Partly because of its longer history and additional notoriety and partly perhaps because of its closeness to the capital (the national news industry remains firmly London-centred), almost any event there is newsworthy. Incidents at the other hospitals are ignored which, if occurring at Broadmoor Hospital, would be national headlines. This is nicely demonstrated by the media coverage of the escape of James Saunders from Broadmoor Hospital in 1992 and of Paul Marshall from Rampton Hospital in 1994. The former occasioned a media circus of the first order while the latter was of relatively minor interest in news terms.

In the summer of 1995 Ashworth Hospital carried out a 'media analysis', comparing the year between June 1994 and May 1995 with the previous years. The analysis made the following key points:

- o In the 12-month period of 1994–5 the analysis of national and local coverage of Ashworth Hospital showed an increase in positive coverage by 15 per cent, while negative coverage remained more or less constant (see Table 20.1).

- o The sharp decline in negative coverage between 1992–3 and 1993–4 was attributable to the high volume of negative stories generated in the earlier year by the Ashworth Inquiry and the reaction to its report.

- o Much of the negative coverage in 1993–4 was due to reporting of the illicit drugs problem at Ashworth, allegations of over-medication of women patients, union statements about increase in danger for staff and a variety of incidents such as ward fires. Negative coverage for 1994–95 was due to the hostage situation on Owen Ward, patient rehabilitation trips, staff evictions, an absconsion from home leave and other small news stories.

- o The rise in positive coverage was mainly due to a proactive campaign to place and initiate a variety of positive stories about Ashworth, a strategy particularly successful in the local and regional press. The regional radio and TV coverage during 1994–95 revealed an equal amount of positive and negative stories, compared with a majority of negative stories in 1993–94.

- o National press coverage tended to be more negative from the tabloid newspapers, but there was a substantial amount of positive national coverage from various gardening magazines, *Refuge, The Big Issue, Lancashire Life*, and Housing Association magazines (a great deal due to a project linked to one housing association). The national professional trade journals also featured some positive articles.

This survey demonstrates what can be achieved through a persistent and well-organised campaign but it is successful principally on a local basis. National at-

Table 20.1 Analysis of press coverage of Ashworth Hospital

1992–3		1993–4		1994–5	
Positive	95	Positive	147	Positive	169
Negative	397	Negative	113	Negative	117
Ratio: 5:1 negative to positive		1.3:1 positive to negative		1.4:1 positive to negative	

Source: Williamson 1995.

tention is more difficult to focus and TV, the eye inside the hospital, presents particular challenges.

In 1993 in Rampton Hospital an arrangement was made with Central TV to film within the walls, the aim being to give a balanced account of the work of the hospital. Included within the itinerary of the TV crew – and carefully planned in advance – was a visit to Anston Ward where some of the most disturbed and exacting of the women patients were resident. Unfortunately, during the filming, the TV crew were left unaccompanied. They learnt that Beverley Allitt was one of the patients and took extensive film of her. From their point of view this was a scoop. For the hospital it was a disaster. A project that started as an attempt to present the hospital in the round degenerated into a legal squabble trying to prevent the film being shown. That failed and the programme when broadcast was, of course, largely concentrated on that one patient. With the predictable emphasis that the media have honed, relatives of her victims relived their anguish on the screen and their cry was 'why is she living in comfort after what she's done?'. This cry overrode any consideration of the hospital's role. It was largely our own fault since we had failed to follow our own guidance by not getting a written agreement in advance of filming and had, additionally, left the crew unsupervised. As a result, relationships between the hospital and TV companies were soured, the PR manager lost his job; and we had failed to protect our patients from intrusion as we had pledged ourselves to do.

The philosophy of openness has to be pursued carefully and cautiously in our world to avoid 'stories' becoming exploitation. Our considered approach made progress. The special hospitals want to remain accessible to the media; they are ready to share purpose, success and failure but they won't do that at the expense of individuals.

SETTING THE RECORD STRAIGHT

Most public institutions will feel that reporting by the media seldom does them justice. In the field of mental health care, there is probably rather more justification for such an attitude. As Doctors Barnes and Earnshaw reported in 1993 on their survey of two daily newspapers' stories on mental illness:

> ...we found that the mentally ill were portrayed almost exclusively in a negative light, with no positive images at all in the tabloid paper. Both papers tended to report the mentally ill conforming to obvious stereotypes. Patients suffering from psychotic illness were presented as violent criminals, committing murder or rape. Those suffering from non-psychotic illnesses were figures of fun, more to be pitied or laughed at than understood.

In the vast majority of cases the tabloid newspaper reported in a sensationalist style, and large print 'banner' headlines were often used. In a number of cases these were actually misleading as to the content of the report (Rapist fools docs with 'I'm mad' plea).

With the Special Hospitals service these responses are even more marked. Given the public apprehension about the combination of mental illness and violence and the media's short-term and shorthand reporting (allowing little opportunity for the balanced consideration of genuinely difficult issues) descriptions of the hospitals and their work are predictably skewed. The distorting mirror held by the media prevails, not just in the national papers but also on TV – a 'Newsnight' report on Rampton Hospital by the BBC in 1991 started with shots of the hospital walls seen through a convenient mist, establishing a 'Hammer' horror atmosphere immediately.

The Press Complaints Commission (PCC) does have a written code, voluntarily agreed by the press industry and ratified in October 1993 which specifically condemns articles and reports which ridicule or distort mental illness:

Discrimination

The press should avoid prejudicial or pejorative reference to a person's race, colour, religion, sex or sexual orientation or to any physical or mental illness or handicap. (Clause 15 (i))

It further defends privacy (N.B. the 'public interest' defence):

Privacy

Intrusions and enquiries into an individual's private life without his or her consent, including the use of long-lens photography to take pictures of people on private property without their consent, are not generally acceptable and publication can only be justified when in the public interest. (Clause 4 (ii))

and makes particular reference to hospitals:

Hospitals

1. Journalists or photographers making enquiries at hospitals or similar institutions should identify themselves to a responsible official and obtain permission before entering non-public areas.

2. The restrictions on intruding into privacy are particularly relevant to enquiries about individuals in hospitals or similar institutions. (Clause 6 (i) and (ii))

This standard was reinforced in February 1994 when the PCC issued an editorial letter to all newspapers advising them on the inappropriateness of prison terminology when describing the work of Special Hospitals:

Editorial: special hospitals and their patients

Since the Mental Health Act 1959 inmates at special hospitals (Rampton, Ashworth, Carstairs and Broadmoor) are designated as 'patients' rather than 'prisoners'. While many such patients are convicted criminals, a number have not committed any crime and their detention for treatment does not stem from an appearance in court. The staff serve in a medical capacity and are not prison officers, although part of their function is to maintain security and they may be members of the Prison Officers' Association.

On a number of occasions since its inception, the Commission has received complaints about the way in which those people in special hospitals are described by the press. In particular, reports of two such complaints by The Matthew Trust, a mental health reform group concerned with issues related to the mentally disordered in secure environments, have been published by the Commission in January and December 1993 (Reports 15, p.6 and 21, p.6). Although neither complaint was upheld because the newspapers involved had taken remedial action, the Commission criticised the inappropriate use of the word 'prisoner' rather than 'patient' in each case.

The Commission reminds editors to ensure that their staff are aware of the classifications of the Mental Health Act 1959 and to take care not to describe special hospitals and their patients in terms which may be considered to breach Clause 1 of the Code of Practice[2].

A revision to the Code was issued in November 1996. There are minor alterations in the section dealing with privacy which have the effect of placing more emphasis on the 'public interest' angle.

Despite these published guidelines, the national press largely still offer the same prejudiced and distorted views that have always been prevalent. There is a marked difference in tone between the tabloids and the broadsheets although the latter can also offer distortions as with *The Times* headline in 1993 'Drugs Take Jail Close to Anarchy' and the *Independent* in March 1996 referring on its front page to 'Broadmoor Prison'. The tabloid stories, however, virtually without exception, feed prejudice and fear usually pressing strongly the buttons marked 'beast' and 'monster', identifying patients as sub or non-human. As, for instance, was illustrated in a story featured in the *Daily Star* on January 26 1996. Under the headline: 'Nutters in beef boycott' they printed the following:

---

2 Clause 1 refers to 'accuracy' of reporting.

The Daily Star has drawn up a helpful menu for the folk who live in Ashworth. It should make a change from nutty cutlets and stir fry.

ASHWORTH MENU

Breakfast
Grapefruit Seg-mentals
Corn Flakeys
Honeynut Loopies

Lunch
Chicken in a Basket-case
Lancashire Hot-potty
Bread and Nutter Pudding

Dinner
Chicken Vinda-loony
Mad Cow Pie

Desserts
Fruitcakes
Spotted Dickhead
Cheese and Crackers

Drinks
I-think-I'm-Napoleon Brandy
A Slow Comfortable Screwed-up.

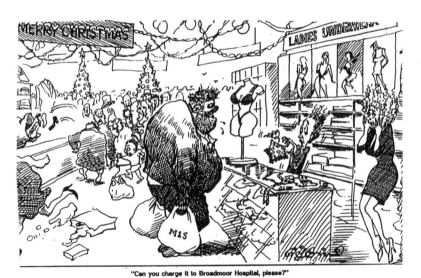

"Can you charge it to Broadmoor Hospital, please?"

Figure 20.3
Source: Daily Mirror, Friday, December 17, 1993

Or as the editor of one national newspaper wrote in 1994 to the general manager of Broadmoor Hospital: 'Truly it is a world going mad when we have to refer to a murderous criminal like Ronnie Kray as a patient'.

Of course the circulation of the tabloids is enormous and six times as large as that of the broadsheets.[3] Every week there is a lot of reinforcement of the negative taking place.

This phenomenon is curiously reinforced by the behaviour of a small minority of the hospitals' staff who persistently and deliberately leak information to the press. Whether this is for cash or reflects dissatisfaction with the changing policies inside the hospital is not clear. It reflects that national ambivalence already noted. Regrettably it is a regular occurrence and efforts to track down those 'moles' have been fruitless. In 1993 Broadmoor Hospital took the Independent News Service to judicial review in an attempt to get them to reveal their 'source' with regard to a particular story. This application was dramatically unsuccessful attracting much criticism and it made clear that legal avenues were unlikely to be helpful in this respect. Interestingly, the action raised three difficult issues. Firstly, press freedom – were we attempting to 'muzzle' the press by trying to prevent them from publishing material we didn't want to see made public? Secondly, the obligations of staff – details given by patients for the purpose of treatment were confidential and should not be shared with the media. Thirdly, staff's freedom to 'blow the whistle'. Our target was to identify the source or 'mole' within the hospital which was giving the press personal details about patients. Undoubtedly, in the legal action and accompanying publicity the hospital was cast as the villain and the news agency as the heroic defender of the right to publish. An important lesson was painfully learnt in trying to change media coverage.

A further lesson arose from the *Sun* story in July 1995 about the move of Ian Brady between different parts of the Ashworth Hospital site. His new location offered an enterprising photographer (no doubt guided by a 'mole'), an opportunity to take a hazy photograph with a telephoto lens (probably from the motorway nearby). We objected formally to this story as an invasion of privacy (ref. Press Complaints Commission code). Both the paper's editor and then the PCC rejected this complaint saying information about this patient was in the domain of public interest. This view was later confirmed in the High Court when Mr Justice Jowitt, in rejecting leave for a judicial review of the PCC ruling, commented:

> It seems to me one has to look at the photographs in the context of the articles they were intended to illustrate, and one has to look at the type of readership the articles are directed at.

3   ABC certified net sale, January 1996: Tabloids 11.086m; Broadsheets 1.736m.

> I do not mean by this that in the tabloid press anything goes. It seems to me it is open to anyone to take the view that the purpose of the photographs is to make the point to the reader that the article, correctly or mistakenly, is appearing to make about the conditions in which Brady is kept.

We made a number of formal complaints to the PCC with mixed success indeed. The response by the paper even to an adjudication in our favour was on occasion less than satisfactory. The *Sunday Mirror* on 19 June 1994 carried an extremely exaggerated story about an incident in Ashworth Hospital headed 'DRUG WAR RIOT IN HOSPITAL'. After correspondence with the paper, we complained to the PCC who ruled against the newspaper. On 29 March 1995, the paper printed the adjudication under the headline 'WE DIDN'T GET IT RIOT'. One assumes that the impact of this 'apology' was marginal, probably only serving to reinforce the original story. An analysis of those complaints submitted and rejected seems to indicate that complaints focusing on individuals are unlikely to succeed; the more profitable ground relates to general principles. Interestingly the fierce public reaction following the death in August of Diana, Princess of Wales (who incidentally visited all of the special hospitals), may accelerate changes in the code and the definition of privacy. While the relationship of the Princess to the media was certainly ambivalent, the circumstances of her death have brought sharply into people's consciousness the intrusive nature of media attention. What is more it has brought media figures out into the open:

> The proven appetite of the public, even the supposedly upmarket public, for sensational personality journalism is huge. Every newspaper in Britain save the Financial Times has moved downmarket, vastly increasing its output of trivia. This is what sells, and we are all dependent on sales to pay our wages.

> We need to stamp out the awful excesses of some parts of the British press, but the chief forces in achieving this will be commercial pressures. (Max Hastings, Editor of the *Evening Standard*, in leading article on 8 September 1997)

The public's indignation may provide that pressure by their frank disapproval which arises from a public tragedy. Ironically that may benefit another section of the community for whom they would probably have little sympathy – the residents of the Special Hospitals.

SUMMING UP

Like most public bodies today, we wanted to be more open about our organisation, its successes and its failures. Indeed we saw such sharing as a positive part of our drive to reduce our hospitals' isolation. We accepted also that investigative journalism had a legitimate role in identifying bad practices within the hospitals. We might prefer that such revelations were not handled sensationally but recognised the value of some of the information that was thus gathered. Some such stories, however, were based on damaging distortions and half-truths. The media's lens can distort as well as reflect; it can burn as well as reveal. Newspapers, and television, can reinforce prejudice and fear (see the review of this subject in Philo 1996) rather than do the more difficult job of explaining risks and dilemmas. We were successful in describing standards and codes of behaviour with regard to the media, successful partially in influencing local reporting but made little positive impact on the national scene. That is unlikely to change until, and unless, the whole attitude towards mental illness is better informed, more tolerant and less frightened.

REFERENCES

Barnes, R.C. and Earnshaw, S. (1993) 'Mental illness in Britain's newspapers'. *Psychiatric Bulletin 17,* 673–674.

Philo, G. (1996) *Media and Mental Distress.* London: Longman.

CHAPTER 21

Criminal Justice System

Jim Higgins

INTRODUCTION

The role of a clinician in a special hospital is a difficult one. It straddles the health service and the criminal justice system, and provides clinical care with simultaneous security for the patient, fellow patients, staff and the general public. The patients are the most difficult to treat and the most dangerous in the country; the number of skilled colleagues is clearly sub-optimal; the hospitals are to a degree professionally, managerially and geographically isolated, semi-detached from other psychiatric services; and there is persistent and intrusive scrutiny of clinical and administrative decisions by external agencies such as Courts, the Home Office, Mental Health Review Tribunals, internal and public inquiries, special interest groups such as WISH (Women in Special Hospitals), the press and others. In crude paraphrase of Dr Johnson it is not that those working in Special Hospitals perhaps do it badly, it sometimes seems remarkable that they do it at all.

Ashworth, Broadmoor and Rampton Hospitals, the three Special Hospitals, are major components of the services for mentally abnormal offenders in England and Wales. Together they currently provide approximately 1500 beds for individuals detained under at least one of the four categories of mental disorder in the Mental Health Act 1983: 67 per cent mental illness, 26 per cent psychopathic disorder, 5 per cent mental impairment and 2 per cent severe mental impairment. The patients have usually been convicted of the most serious offences but not all are detained as a result of an appearance in court. A quarter have been transferred from another psychiatric facility following disturbed and dangerous behaviour without criminal charges having been brought. Three quarters of the patients are male. The length of stay of a patient can be as short as a few months for assessment of suitability for treatment but it may be a lifetime for a small number of the persistently very dangerous. The average length of stay is more than seven years but such a figure reveals little, an arithmetical artefact which disguises the very particular circumstances of a large number of virtually unique individuals.

Patients admitted to Special Hospitals come either from other psychiatric services or from various aspects of the criminal justice system but the degree to which the special hospitals, or the criminal lunatic asylums as they were earlier called and the high security hospitals as they are now called, have been integrated into the health or criminal justice system has varied considerably. Until relatively recently, not just the view of the public and many of the staff but the funding and management arrangements and the style and quality of professional practice had served to distance the Special Hospitals from the mainstream not just of general psychiatry, but also from the regional forensic psychiatry services which have been developing throughout England and Wales since the mid 1970s. However, the pressures towards insularity have not all been one way. There have been incentives for general psychiatric services to keep the Special Hospitals and their patients at a distance. The admission of a patient to a Special Hospital for a lengthy period of expensive treatment has been a free good. Issues surrounding a difficult patient could be shelved for years. Closer and more integrated work with Special Hospitals raises theoretical, clinical and politically difficult issues, the question of the proper balance between treatment and control of very difficult individuals, particularly those with major personality disorders, and how, where and in what way this balance could be better struck. Closer involvement of professional organisations only results in the need to confront issues of professional and ethical standards and the enduring difficulties of recruitment in three large and increasingly anachronistic establishments, closer to the criminal justice system than any other health service facility and under more intensive political, administrative and media scrutiny, whether justified or not.

THE 1980S AND BEYOND

In the last 20 years all these features have led to two distinct forensic psychiatry systems. Regional forensic psychiatry services are based on regional secure units which are small and integrated with local psychiatric and social services. They are well staffed and without major recruitment problems and accommodate patients whose length of stay is not intended to exceed two years. High security hospitals are large secure institutions which usually have difficulties in recruiting and retraining psychiatrists, psychologists and more recently nursing staff sufficient for their needs. Daunting case-loads serve to obstruct the development of effective multidisciplinary working which in any event was rarely the traditional style of working.

It is observations like these which have led to demands that Special Hospitals must change, even to the extent that some consider that their liabilities are so ingrained that they must be closed and alternative arrangements made. The first recent and major attempt to change the way Special Hospitals were administered, run and managed was by the formation of the Special Hospitals Service Authority in 1989. This resulted in the disbandment of the role of the medical directors with managerial and clinical responsibility for the hospitals and the introduction of general management. As a result of the changes made, and on the advice of The Working Group on High Security and Related Psychiatric Provision (Reed II) which reported in 1994, a modified version of the purchaser / provider model was introduced as in the rest of the health service. The High Security Psychiatric Services Commissioning Board (HSPSCB), a national purchasing / commissioning authority, was eventually set up and each high security hospital became a Special Hospital Authority with freedom to manage its internal affairs independently, akin to but not identical to an NHS Trust hospital. The commissioning role is still evolving. The intention is to restrict the admission to a high security hospital to only those patients requiring high security and to develop forensic psychiatry services elsewhere to cater for patients who require longer-term secure care but do not require high security. The isolation of the hospitals and their staff is to be reduced by better integration into the other forensic services and the perverse incentive of a free place in a high security hospital is eventually to be removed. Academic links have already been fostered and a Chair of Special Hospital Psychiatry has been founded at Broadmoor Hospital.

The purchasing strategy to be developed will be driven by an assessment of the treatment and security needs of each patient and where these might best be met. The plan is that this needs assessment and the funding of its implementation will be taken over by those at a more local level who are already responsible for purchasing existing regional forensic and general psychiatry services. Care will however need to be taken to ensure that such fragmentation of funding will not result in current monies being dissipated. There will probably remain a need for a degree of national and regional strategic planning and oversight.

If this strategy is successful the High Security Hospitals Service should probably not exceed 800–1000 beds but it is as yet unclear where these beds should be sited: in all three hospitals, in fewer, or dispersed in smaller units elsewhere integrated into relevant local services. Even if the last solution is preferred there will still remain the challenge of treating and managing patients who require high security, particularly those with serious intractable mental illness or those with serious personality disorder either alone or in association with an additional mental illness.

The extent of this challenge should not be underestimated. This challenge has become much greater since the introduction of increased legal rights for patients, the expectation of more individual and more liberal treatment plans and the consequent greater difficulty in balancing individual treatment needs with the flexible complex arrangements required to meet these with vigilance and security often of a high order and over a very lengthy period of time. Patients and their advocates are now more demanding. Scrutiny by the Home Office, the Department of Health, the Mental Health Act Commission, Mental Health Review Tribunals, the SHSA and its successor the HSPSCB, is more intense, magnified by the unfortunate tendency of recent politicians, driven by the press or factional interests, to rush to the formation of committees of inquiry whenever something untoward happens. The pressure of all of this perhaps explains why recruitment of most types of staff is difficult and why those who do choose to work in such a setting and under such pressure decide after a period of time or after a set of circumstances that life is more congenial elsewhere. It is almost certainly naive to expect that if such high-profile and professionally demanding patients were relocated elsewhere the pressures would be much less, but working in a more integrated and supportive and less isolated environment might make them more tolerable and perhaps even stimulating.

INFLUENCE OF THE CRIMINAL JUSTICE SYSTEM

So what are the professional challenges confronting those working in high security settings and to a degree those working in other forensic psychiatry settings?

By far the majority of patients in high security hospitals are detained under Part III of the Mental Health Act 1983, those sections dealing with mentally abnormal offenders. A few have been found unfit to plead and even fewer guilty by reason of insanity. The remainder are technically non-offenders detained under Part II of the Act (Section 3) yet also dangerous patients in need of long-term treatment.

Part III of the Act has a variety of provisions to enable the detention of an individual for assessment and treatment at various stages of progression through the criminal justice system. There is a group of sections which empower a court to order the assessment or treatment of an individual in a hospital before sentence: Section 35, a remand for a (psychiatric) report; Section 36, a remand for treatment; Section 38, a remand of a convicted defendant for a lengthy assessment to explore the wisdom of a Hospital Order, particularly when treatability in hospital is the principle issue. The Hospital Order, Section 37, a simple hospital order, is the principle psychiatric disposal of a court. This results in admission to and detention in hospital. This detention is reviewed after six months and thereafter at yearly intervals and can be contested by the patient at similar intervals by an Appeal to Managers (of the hospital) or more usually by an application to a Mental Health Review Tribunal. However, as most patients in secure hospitals have committed a serious violent offence, the trial judge, after verbal psychiatric evidence, will have imposed an additional order, a Restriction Order, Section 41, which removes from the responsible medical officer, the consultant in charge of the patient's care, and from the managers, the ability to transfer or discharge the patient. Only the Home Secretary can do both; a Mental Health Review Tribunal can only do the latter.

Some patients, also detained under Part III of the Act, are transferred to hospital without the intervention of a court. These are remanded prisoners in need of urgent treatment, transferred under Section 48 almost invariably with an additional Section 49 (the restriction direction, analogous to Section 41), or sentenced prisoners in need of urgent treatment transferred under Section 47 and Section 49. At the end of periods of treatment sentenced prisoners / patients will return to prison but may remain in hospital after the expiry of their sentence if their psychiatric condition mandates this. In exceptional circumstances a few may be discharged as if they had initially been detained under Sections 37/41. As many Section 47/49 patients are serving life sentences, mandatory or discretionary, there is cross-referral to the Parole Board with consequent complexity.

The above brief and simplified account of relevant aspects of the Mental Health Act is complicated enough but it does no justice to the volume and detail of the work required of a responsible medical officer and his or her colleagues throughout an individual patient's contact with a high security hospital or other secure hospital. The particular characteristics of the patients and what they have done and the need for regular involvement of Courts, the Home Office, Mental Health Review Tribunals and other interested parties regularly raise clinical, organisational and ethical issues not often encountered in general psychiatric practice. Such regular scrutiny of practice by outside agencies demands much time-consuming report and letter writing in an atmosphere which may be adversarial. A description of how a hypothetical patient is considered for admission, is admitted for treatment, is then subsequently managed and is ultimately prepared for transfer or discharge will highlight these areas of work.

ADMISSION PROCESS

A consultant from a Special Hospital will usually be approached about a potential patient by a psychiatrist working in local general psychiatry services, local forensic psychiatry services or in prison. The referral might also be made directly by a defendant's solicitor who feels that the expertise of a Special Hospital consultant is required or that a placement in a high security hospital needs to be explored. The initial assessment has to be made in the setting where the patient is placed, a local psychiatric hospital, local secure unit or in prison. This assessment needs to be comprehensive not just because of the complexity of medico-legal issues usually involved but the difficulties in estimating risk and the exact level of security which may be required. The assessment is undertaken by the consultant allocated to the case and usually also by a nursing member of the multidisciplinary team within which both work. A forensic clinical psychologist and a social worker, also members of the team, may also be involved. If the request is solely for a risk assessment or a second opinion on treatment a written opinion will be provided but if, as is more usual, the request for the assessment was but a forerunner to a request for an admission to a high security hospital, then a written report plus supporting documentation must be provided to the admissions panel of the special hospital. The membership of the admissions panel and its procedures are slightly different in the three hospitals but each considers the assessment report and all the referral material and then either declines to admit the patient or agrees to an admission for further assessment or for longer-term treatment.

Admissions panels are rarely found elsewhere in psychiatric practice as they are seen as archaic or an infringement of the clinical freedom of a consultant. They have traditionally been felt necessary in high security hospitals, first by the Department of Health and then by the SHSA who controlled admissions. This function has in recent years been devolved to the hospitals themselves and it is still felt to be necessary to set criteria for admission to scarce high security beds and to resist the often considerable pressures for admission of inappropriate referrals. Occasionally, the rejection of a referral can cause disappointment to a court, the Home Office, to other psychiatric services and even to an assessing Special Hospital consultant and the colleagues who made the assessment and recommended admission.

Two groups of patients raise the most difficulty in assessment for admission, those with severe personality disorders and those with a chronic mental illness which results in behaviour which requires management in a moderately secure setting and for an expected very lengthy period.

The treatability of those with a severe personality disorder is a very contentious issue. There is almost as much difference of view amongst Special Hospital consultants as there is elsewhere, though there are some notable enthusiasts. The willingness to accept such patients is currently quite different in the three hospitals. Even if admission is further restricted there will remain a substantial cohort of seriously personality disordered patients who have been in hospital for many years and whose poor response to treatment indicates that they will not be ready for discharge or transfer for very many years, or ever. For those with a severe chronic mental illness associated with continuing risk of violence, the availability of local lower security facilities varies considerably in the catchment area of the three Special Hospitals, and this has had an influence on the referral rates of such patients to each of the hospitals and on the expectation that such patients will be admitted. In recent years increasing care has had to be taken to ensure that the need for medium security over a long period does not result in admission to high security as unfortunately it has in the past.

After an admission for further assessment or for a protracted period of treatment a detailed initial assessment of what are inevitably very complex patients is required. This may or may not be done in a specialist admission unit. Those patients already well known to psychiatric services will have been referred not just because of the degree of immediate risk but because of a longer history of disturbed behaviour, arising from mental illness which has proved resistant to conventional treatment. A careful analysis needs to be undertaken of previous patterns of behaviour and its antecedents, and relevant personality factors, and a review made of response to various types of medication prescribed in the past. A multidisciplinary care plan can then be drawn up to meet the needs of the patient within a context which ensures the safety of the patient, other patients and staff.

Patients coming from the criminal justice system may or may not have had previous contact with psychiatric services but will often be known to social services, the probation service, the penal system. Despite the careful pre-admission assessment there is usually considerable additional information to be obtained before arriving at a preliminary view of the relative importance of mental illness, personality characteristics, substance abuse and other factors, all of which are often present to varying degrees in mentally abnormal offenders who commit the most serious offences and who pose the greatest risk. An assessment of the interplay of these factors is essential to decide which are to be dealt with first and to ensure that important features which might become less prominent during a lengthy stay in a secure and controlling environment do not get forgotten.

Treatment planning and its implementation is therefore complex, highly multidisciplinary and strategic – or it should be, but individual case-loads, shortage of skilled staff, changes of key staff, limited flexibility in hospitals which are invariably full, security considerations which are rightly or wrongly considered paramount and traditional staff attitudes can easily result in discrepancies between what is required and what can be provided. The introduction of the Care Programme Approach has been difficult and patchy in psychiatry as a whole. The high security hospitals are no different; however, the complexities of the clinical, administrative and legal issues make such a strategic clinical approach even more necessary but at the same time more difficult to achieve in the setting of a large hospital whose patients can come from distant parts of the country, stay for a very long time and are often looked after by a series of multi-disciplinary teams in circumstances which are not ideal.

PATIENTS' RIGHTS

Most patients in Special Hospitals contest their detention and question their treatment. They do this to a degree not seen elsewhere, even in other secure psychiatric settings. This is their legal right and it is quite proper that they do. This contesting and questioning is no doubt a reflection of the length of detention and of the seeming powerlessness of patients, and perhaps also of staff, to move a case on when this seems clinically appropriate. Scrutiny of risk factors by the Home Office sometimes results in lengthy delays and differences of opinion. An application to a Mental Health Review Tribunal is therefore a way of testing issues of treatment and detention and of gauging the Home Office view even when conditional discharge is untimely and grossly unlikely on clinical grounds or estimate of risk or both.

While such applications are often driven by the patients themselves it sometimes seems as if there is an MHRT industry, fuelled by legal aid, legal representation and the ready availability of independent medical opinions often of those not regularly involved in the practice of forensic psychiatry. An adversarial climate can easily be engendered and some high-profile MHRTs are highly adversarial with all parties represented by counsel. These can have deleterious effects on staff morale and the therapeutic alliance between the patients and their carers. On the other hand this audit of the performance of the clinical team and the review of progress can have the beneficial effects of suggesting new approaches or highlighting unavailability of resources, though, sadly, not of providing the resources. The recommendation of a MHRT can only be to discharge or not to discharge a patient. It cannot order a transfer to another hospital setting with lower security or even no security and if the Home Office has previously objected to such a move, a hearing in favour of such a proposal can often lead to lingering dissatisfaction and frustration in the patient and the staff.

THE ROLE OF THE HOME OFFICE

The Home Office requires annual statutory reports on all restricted patients. These are requested by the Mental Health Division, the department responsible for all but the clinical management of restricted patients in hospitals. It is also responsible for large numbers of conditionally discharged patients in the community. The Mental Health Division is staffed exclusively by civil servants. There are 4250 restricted patients in hospitals and 1500 conditionally discharged patients overseen by 50 staff, eight senior staff, 28 case workers and 14 clerical staff. The remit of the Mental Health Division is to advise the Home Secretary (in practice a Minister of State at the Home Office) on the transfer or discharge of restricted patients. As the ultimate responsibility of the Minister is public safety, and the political presentation of this, rather than the clinical care of a patient, it is inevitable and proper that the Home Office takes a cautious and questioning stance, requiring that all relevant risk factors have been identified and dealt with to a degree which makes the risk of onward movement acceptable and defensible. It would therefore be surprising if there was always unanimity of view between the Home Office and the multidisciplinary team caring for a patient.

Most cases proceed relatively smoothly, particularly those who suffer from a serious mental illness which has played the predominant part in the commission of their dangerous behaviour, and who have shown steady improvement in their condition with appropriate medication. Other factors such as substance misuse can be tackled and after a period of initial consolidation and improvement, which might last some years, the Home Office can readily be engaged in a plan of increasing escorted leave from the hospital and in discussions about eventual transfer to a hospital offering a lower degree of security, such as a regional secure unit.

The Home Office will probably initially agree to a period of trial leave in lower security prior to formal transfer, but only when it feels comfortable with the expectation that the patient is then likely to be conditionally discharged to the community within two years. The direction of travel of such cases is rarely in doubt though the rate of progress may be disputed. The Home Office is more likely to agree to a proposal when all relevant factors including the likely political perception have been acknowledged at the outset and plans made for the treatment or management of each factor with critical evaluation of success. Regular contact over a planned series of gradual steps is a much more successful means of communicating and working together than more sudden leaps or changes of direction driven by factors which cannot easily be identified or evaluated.

Pressures from patients or their advocates for transfer or discharge can be considerable, either quite overt or quietly persistent over a long period of time, and these can sometimes lead to a view of a case by some or all of the multidisciplinary team which from a more distant, uninvolved and perhaps cynical perspective seems flawed and even risky.

A particular difficulty can occur in cases where there is multiple serious psychopathology. Marked improvement in one area, such as social skills and an ability to survive harmoniously in the hospital with fellow patients and staff, can lead over a long period to a decreasing awareness that it was, for example, serious sexual psychopathology or arson which was the reason why the patient was admitted in the first place. This is especially likely when attempts to deal with these features were never adequate or took place years before, and when the effectiveness of the interventions cannot be properly evaluated because of a lack of opportunity to repeat the index behaviour in a controlled and secure setting.

Talk of discharge or transfer can easily reactivate Home Office concerns in these areas and lead to questions and requests for further information which to a consultant, who may only have been in charge of the case for at most a few years, can seem impossible to investigate, impossible to answer with the required degree of certainty and just frankly obstructive and procrastinating. Beside the obvious differences of responsibility and interest, and the influences or even distortions which these may produce, it is very difficult or even impossible to make a defensible assessment of risk in some cases, particularly those of individuals with severe personality disorders with sexual psychopathology who were admitted to hospital many years ago and who would now never even be considered for admission.

ADVISORY BOARD

Following the aftermath of the discharge of Graham Young with his subsequent reoffending in a dangerous fashion, when the medical advice was that he was no longer a risk, the Advisory Board on Restricted Patients was formed in 1971 to advise the Home Secretary on the risks of the transfer or discharge of patients who particularly concern him and the civil servants. The Advisory Board, as it is called, has evolved over the intervening years in its remit and its membership. Initially, it was felt that high risk cases could and should be identified at the outset and should be considered by the Advisory Board later on. This proved unrealistic and impractical. Gradually it has become that it is those cases which concern the senior officials of the Mental Health Division which are considered by the Board though the Minister can refer any case, and how often and in what circumstances this is done varies with the Minister. The sorts of cases referred by the officials of the Mental Health Division are those described above: those where risk is multi-factorial; where some of the factors have not been properly identified or addressed; where the results of intervention have been equivocal; where there have been lengthy and unresolved differences of view between the Home Office and all or some members of the multidisciplinary team.

The Board consists of eight members: two legal representatives, one of whom is a judge and is the chairman; two forensic psychiatrists; two 'social workers', usually a chief probation officer and a director of social services; and two lay persons with knowledge of the criminal justice system. Any member of the Board will be asked to visit the hospital where the patient resides, not exclusively a high security hospital, and will interview the patient and the relevant members of the multidisciplinary team. The purpose is not to test the diagnosis, for this would not be appropriate for the non-medical members of the Board, but to test the quality of the information upon which the estimate of risk is being made and the quality of the multidisciplinary consultation and decision-making processes. A brief report is then prepared which accompanies the detailed dossier prepared on each case for a Board meeting. Confidential advice is submitted to the Minister after often lengthy discussion. Despite the Board supporting the majority of discharge and transfer proposals put to it, its function and method of working have come under increasing scrutiny in recent years and the confidentiality of the whole procedure has been questioned. It is likely that legal challenges will continue.

NEXT STEPS

The future of the high security hospitals is under active consideration at the present time. There are pressures to make considerable changes to the roles of the hospitals, even to the extent of considering closing the three existing hospitals and replacing only their high security function in smaller units integrated with the regional forensic psychiatry services which already exist. The difficulties of being a patient in a Special Hospital or of staff working in a Special Hospital argue strongly for major changes but important issues first need to be resolved: whether to continue admitting patients with very severe personality disorders; how to treat them; where to treat them; how to manage humanely those individuals, mostly with a personality disorder, who are unlikely ever to be discharged; how best to provide for smaller groups of patients with special needs such as women, those with marked learning disabilities, those with brain damage. How will a devolved system meet the needs of such a wide range of difficult patients? These questions are no longer a reflection of the isolation of the high security hospitals but result from the changes that they have recently been making. Nor do they arise just from critics on the outside of the hospitals. They were high on the agenda of the SHSA, are high on the agenda of the HSPSCB and are under active discussion by the staff of the three hospitals. Much will now depend on the welcome from local forensic psychiatry services and their willingness to review and amend their policies and practices. Above all, a strong political impetus will be required before high security hospitals can move into the mainstream of psychiatric practice.

PART 6

Summing Up

CHAPTER 22

Achievements and the Future

Charles Kaye and Alan Franey

WORK IN PROGRESS

This book has described a relatively short period of time in the evolution of the high security psychiatric service and of the three hospitals that currently provide that service. It would be presumptuous to claim revolutionary success within those few years; there is a long history which cannot be discarded and a host of contemporary factors, some of which help change while others hinder it.

The testimony gathered together has tried honestly, even if sometimes painfully, to describe what we set out to do in the late 1980s, what devices and techniques we used, and how far we travelled towards our goals. In a real sense every chapter is incomplete because further improvement can be, and is, sought for. Changing large organisations and attempting to influence public opinion presents a pathway where the chicanes of vested interest are almost as fearsome as the pits of prejudice. Sometimes we navigated surely; at other times we stumbled. Overall we strongly believe that we have publicly set new standards and expectations which cannot in the future be ignored.

Although a relaxation of managerial and professional vigilance may allow standards to fall back temporarily in some areas, the aspirations and needs which have been described remain constant.

Some observers may comment that any claims for progress are vitiated by reported episodes of failure within the service or of reoffending outside it. In part this is to fail to understand the nature of these patients and their illnesses. As one former Broadmoor patient, Peter Thompson, described:

Every crime committed by a mentally ill person is a two-fold tragedy, one for the person injured or offended against, and one for the offender. More often than not, the offender, before he or she commits the crime, has been crying out for help from a society too deaf to hear. (quoted in Longford 1992)

The patients are severely mentally ill and the outcomes of treatment and care reflect that: a recent study at Rampton Hospital showed that for a sample of discharged patients: 'Mortality for both men and women was twice that of the population base adjusted for age and the length of follow-up' (Steels *et al.* in press). The difficulties of care, and the risks of discharge, are exacerbated by the pitch of the patient's illness. Most of these patients have passed through other levels of care which proved ineffective and they reach high security almost in desperation, both for themselves and for others who have tried to help.

> Patients requiring high security psychiatric services are likely to suffer from more than one disorder (including physical illnesses) and are more likely than other psychiatric patients to present with multiple diagnoses. Primary diagnosis is thus a crude guide only to the nature of each patient's illness, and we acknowledge that a patient's primary diagnosis will not reflect the full range or combination of clinical conditions that must be addressed. Further, multiple diagnosis sometimes means that during their stay in special hospital a patient's primary diagnosis can change, either as treatment progresses or the patient's condition fluctuates. Added to this is a number of complicating factors such as brain damage, drug abuse, alcohol misuse and sex offending. It is clear, therefore, given the kaleidoscopic nature of patients requiring high security psychiatric services, that it is important that providers avoid over-simplification in their approach to meeting patients' needs. (HSPSCB 1996/1997)

Similarly, failure to meet standards or to apply lessons and techniques learnt is not a telling indictment of management and professional competence, but rather an indication of the magnitude of the task approached.

The manager's view of things as he describes them as they ought to be (and hopefully will be) is always at some distance from the varied reality of how things are – that reality is like an uneven rank with some heads taller. Such a discrepancy will always exist: it is in itself one of the products of, and witnesses to, leadership. Every good manager knows that – it does not make him a hypocrite; but much depends on his keen awareness of how great the disparity is, where it is at its most critical and whether it is increasing or decreasing.

The increments of progress are described but there are more to be achieved.

TOUCHSTONES FOR THE FUTURE

In analysing experience over the lifetime of the SHSA it has been possible to crystallise a small number of simple observations which are crucial to any sympathetic understanding of the present and the future. The following octet provides a set of reference points which should guide commentary on, and planning of, the future of this service. They are valid within the Special Hospitals, but equally applicable to any consideration of high security psychiatric care.

- Number of patients is small; risks and complications huge.
- The service must be defined in terms of patients and their needs, not in terms of facilities provided.
- Security is a key dimension within the definition of patients' needs: but it is erroneous and misleading to use it in isolation as a way of describing patients (e.g. 'High Security Patients' etc.).
- The patient population is clinically heterogeneous: we need more and better descriptions of the variety and differences.
- This is predominantly long-term care with few (if any) cures. Each patient needs one personal plan of care and support to which all relevant agencies subscribe and contribute.
- Forensic psychiatry is frontier medicine and knowledge is patchy and uneven; targeted, well constructed research is essential.
- Each element of service will only be as good as the staff who provide it; better staff will require more focused training and plenty of support.
- It is a collaborative world; patients will probably also be clients, suspects and prisoners. Health alone will not meet their needs.

MANAGEMENT BY RULES

In large organisations it is important to clarify key policies – for understanding and consistency – and often these policies spawn, or even spontaneously mutate into, sets of values. The inquiry climate reinforces this tendency: let's have a set of procedures to ensure this doesn't happen again. The anxiety of politicians and the vulnerability of managers lead them to support this approach. And such is the power of this movement that all involved, including the practitioner next to the patient, can forget the purpose of the rule and simply regard its existence as a self-justifying artifact. Often the presence of procedures or policies has been offered, and taken, as indication that all is well. The SHSA has not been without fault in sometimes focusing on the form at the expense of the substance. A good approach to rules is contained in a nicely described code drawn up by James Willis. He observes that: 'The essential point is that rules can never describe life, they can only set the limits' (Willis 1995). He amplifies this in his 'Rules for Rules':

- Rules should always be implemented properly so that they are respected. If a rule has been made to be broken then it has been made badly.

- Rules must never, ever, be made for their own sake or for the sake of change. It is never right, under any circumstances, for rules to be created as a justification for the existence of the rule makers or to satisfy their need for power, authority and status. Rulemakers should be servants of society, not rulers of society; rules should be instruments of informed consensus.

- Rules must always be practical – which means they will often be far less stringent than we think (– and enormously less stringent than a specialist in the particular field would think).

- The number of rules must be kept to an indispensable minimum – which means there will be far fewer than we think (– and enormously fewer than the sum of all the recommendations of all specialists).

- Rules should always be created and applied at the most peripheral level of society possible. The best rules are imposed by the responsible adult on himself and each step away from this ideal must be justified.

- Rules should be *safe minimum baselines* not *impossible ideals*. They should be foundations on which to build, not mountain-tops people exhaust themselves struggling vainly to reach. People are best left choosing their own mountains to climb.

- Rules should be designed to set the limits of acceptable behaviour, not to direct the details of behaviour.

Or to put it another way: only make rules and guidelines that are essential and put your effort into training and supporting your staff rather than into creating for them a procedural obstacle race.

MARKERS OF PROGRESS

In the high security world it is always important to retain a distinction between the contents and the vessel. The service itself is provided by three large institutions. We do not expect that to continue and describe later in this chapter some of the changes we would propose. However, in the present situation there is an unfortunate – and widespread – tendency to see the service and the hospitals as an indivisible whole. There is often confusion in comments and thinking which reflect the failure of speakers to distinguish between the needs of patients and the limitations of the existing sites. Conversely the hospitals and their staffs are held responsible for problems which are intrinsic to the care of such patients and which can only be avoided if no care is provided – other than in a prison's hospital wing.

In our review of the last decade we have deliberately separated achievements into two classes – those that apply specifically to the Special Hospitals (and thus represent those institutions' rate of progress); and those that apply to the high security service as a whole. This distinction could be characterised as short-term and long-term. There is of course overlap between the two and many service-wide improvements have their impact on the three hospitals.

However, maintaining such a duality is valuable particularly in teasing out key principles for the future.

ACHIEVEMENTS IN THE SPECIAL HOSPITALS

Among a wide range of changes the following seem to us critical:

- Introducing 24-hour care – converting the 'prison by night' into continuous care.
- Eliminating 'slopping out' – the ritualised indignity of denying human beings access to a toilet.
- Emphasising professional standards – the expectations a trained person imposes on him or herself.
- The proper balance between care and custody – as the SHSA expressed it: 'the provision of good basic physical security and associated systems should provide the possibility of a relatively relaxed regime within those boundaries. Efficient security should therefore enhance treatment and provide a safe background against which patients can test out this progress' (SHSA 1992).
- The furtherance of patients' rights – describing what they could expect and their role as partners in care.
- Introducing general management – leadership with a clear chain of command with responsibilities and concomitant authority.
- Revitalising the rehabilitation service – to move from 'occupations', prison-like diversional work, towards specific therapies.
- Academic units – creating professional posts and supporting units in each hospital.
- Improving living conditions – improving the fabric, building new accommodation and removing most of the dormitories.

ADVANCING THE SERVICE

These changes, while focused on or originating in the hospitals, provide key initiatives for the development of a service differently organised in the future:

- Closer integration within the NHS – this will always be a service with strong and proper links to criminal justice but it should be not regarded by the NHS as an alien creature.
- Setting standards and devising methods of measuring progress – bringing in quality in a measurable manner.
- Better description of patients and their needs – moving beyond a security classification towards the clinically specific.

- Bringing training and education to centre-stage.
- Reappraisal of the roles of staff – changes in patterns of training, recruitment and working.
- Drive to reshape the national service – on the basis of need, not bureaucracy.
- Emphasis on well-constructed research and application of its results.
- Closer working with prisons.

These themes reappear in our views about the future.

UNRESOLVED ISSUES

Although it is acknowledged that most of the above advances still have further to go, it is worth pointing out some areas where the struggle has been intense and efforts should be redoubled. Two are specific to the Special Hospitals (the first two points in the list) while the others apply throughout the mental health service:

- Changing the culture – the negative attitudes, so often commented on, have been pushed back but not eliminated. Rather like a cultivated garden, if the weeds are not quickly removed they can soon dominate. The situation is much improved but needs constant monitoring and attention.
- The POA – this union has consistently acted as a focus for custodians and as an opponent of change. It epitomises the 'turnkey tradition'. It should have no place in a care-orientated setting.
- Racial and gender awareness – while much of the overt prejudice is no longer evident (although it may perhaps just have gone underground) there is an evident need for progress towards a better understanding of difference and prejudice – and the application of such understanding to care and treatment.
- Multidisciplinary work – team-working is universally preached and superficially accepted. It remains in practice an elusive chimera. Professional training and public criticism inhibit its development. Team-working is still concentrated more on what staff *do* than on what patients *need*.
- Support and preparation of staff. Management still does not do enough to help staff to be effective. Training is spasmodic and often random in its focus. Support systems for staff working in the most difficult clinical situations are still in their infancy. The rule of thumb for judging staff effectiveness is still 'how many', rather than 'how capable'.

THE FUTURE

Principles

Two misapprehensions above all bedevil clear thought about the future requirements for high security psychiatric care. First, there is confusion between the service, the patients and their requirements, and the special hospitals themselves. The latter are the current repository of the service; their advantages and drawbacks should not become – as is so often the case – the currency for describing the future. Undoubtably they circumscribe the present and will be a major component in the near future but they are not definitively and indefinitely the service. Second, there is the too readily accepted divide between different levels of security. Thus the medium secure units exist almost in a different world where connections with high security units are difficult and uneasy and always to the detriment of the patient.

No comprehensive secure service is at present available in England and Wales; rather there is an archipelago of semi-autonomous clinical units masquerading as a continent. We see a collection of fiefdoms sharing little interest in life outside their own boundaries, as if their own separate existence was self-justifying.

To remedy these astigmatic defects, we consider that any plans for change, for the future, must start with carefully considered principles against which rearrangements should continually be measured. Our principles follow.

Integration
In secure psychiatric care there should be one service with different levels of security catered for in a manner which supports patient care, and a flexibility in response to patients' improvements and decline, which avoids the snakes and ladders approach of the current system. We must shed a system devised for the convenience of bureaucrats or doctors.

Cohesive Management
Whatever management pattern is adopted must facilitate such integration and enable patients to move quickly according to clinical needs and without penalty. It should be based on paths, not boundaries. Similarly, financial dispositions must mirror the management pattern. This does not mean special hospital 'dowries' which are a short-term device to overcome present divisions. We need a financing system which takes in its accounting stride the regular movement of patients between different units, both NHS and private, and removes the financial camouflage under which reluctant managers and clinicians shelter to avoid patients they do not want to accommodate.

Specific Services
What is to be provided must be based on a full analysis of the needs of identifiable homogenous groups of patients. At present we regard patients in bulk,

eliminating or ignoring key differences and shoehorning them into what is ar-
bitrarily available. To be better we must be more specific and consider the realities we know exist. Such future distinctions need proper debate but will
probably include:

- gender-specific – women
- function-specific – assessment
- age – adolescent
- diagnostic – learning disability, personality disorder

The key starting point will be a nationally arranged assessment service (as in
Holland), with designated centres where a clinical evaluation takes place which
sets the tone for treatment, moves the patient to the most appropriate location
and presents clinical consistency. Security and dependence will no longer be
absolutes in describing facilities but become requirements which fluctuate in
each patient's career and therefore will be provided according to his or her
needs.

Staffing and Training

There is a dismally low regard paid to the key requirement of finding the right
people and giving them the most appropriate training. Much talk but little action. Again and again the real problems of treating patients with severe psychiatric illness, usually chronic, often dangerous, are compounded by not having
the right staff for a very difficult job. The conventional professional distinctions
as often impede care as progress it with individuals as interested in professional
dignity (roles) as in contributing (skills). The intractability of team-working
demonstrates this continually.

We need a new approach to recruitment (proper profiling, no 'unqualified'
staff); to training (targeted specifically towards the needs and demands of the
different groups of patients); to movement of staff (to avoid 'burn-out' and to
prevent them getting locked into one location or institution); and to the make-
up of the staff team (there should be vigorous testing of the 'social therapist'
model since today's student nurses are clearly demonstrating that psychiatric
nursing is an unattractive career option).

Particularly with training and the standards of education, this suggests some
national overview. Individual local efforts are unco-ordinated, often duplicate
each other and lack consistent standards. More training and more focused
training is a key message and one far more important than new buildings.

Research and Development

Research and development must underpin progress of the service, test new hypotheses and spread evidence, and encourage adoption of successful practice.
This is not to stifle innovation but to accelerate learning. A national research

programme is needed which is specific to secure psychiatric care, truly multidisciplinary, and has the proper apparatus for scrutiny and dissemination.

Prisons and Probation

Any changes to the secure psychiatric services must take into account the existence and problems of the criminal justice system, in particular the courts and prisons. The realities of patients' illnesses and behaviour means that many, probably most, will be prisoners as well. A proper service must recognise this and devise ways of crossing yet more frontiers where opposing groups of public servants bat disadvantaged individuals backwards and forwards in avoidance. Initiatives should be developed together.

Size

Institutions (existing or new) should not be too large. The larger they are, the more difficult they are to manage and the more problematic it is to ensure that the culture and behaviour of staff reflects the values publicly declared, rather than a silent but powerful counter culture. There are no absolute figures but it is unlikely that locations offering more than 200 beds or employing more than 500 staff will be culturally and clinically consistent. While many will see this as a direct comment on the special hospitals, it would be as well to recognise that new institutions are developing, as 'successful' Trusts accrete a range of services on one site.

National Scrutiny

Such a service should continually be under a national microscope. Its very importance and the attendant continual risks necessitate public confidence; its high costs require demonstration of value for money. The present *ad hoc* scrutiny in retrospect, by a series of unco-ordinated inquiries, is unhelpful and indifferently organised with no consistent criteria and little demonstrable benefit.

We propose the creation of a national body for planning and developing the service, using well thought-out criteria, and also the introduction of a scrutinising organisation which inspects and judges. The latter body should have the power to license organisations and locations to provide secure psychiatric care; its ultimate sanction would be the withdrawal of a licence. It too would operate according to published criteria and would publish its regular reviews. It could assimilate, or build upon, the work of the Mental Health Act Commission.

Conclusion

Adopting these principles – or variations upon them – would mark the creation of a service which truly was national in scope and patient-centred in outlook: two characteristics notably absent today. It would herald national standards in training, research and service provision together with a national licensing body reviewing *all* providers. (Incidentally it is appropriate to emphasise that 'national' does not, in our eyes, equate with 'Departmental'. Richmond House (or Wellington House) has a contribution to make, but 'national' means 'incorporating the best of all available knowledge and practice').

The service would be various to accommodate different needs at present ignored. It would have a funnel – through assessment centres – which would aid clinical consistency and simplify access to the service at all levels. There would be more specialisation but also far more flexibility and an acceptance of the need to demonstrate effectiveness both in terms of clinical practice and expenditure.

In such a context the vexed question of personality disorder and its 'treatability' could be approached using medical knowledge, science and experience rather than prejudice or expediency. A national service could introduce and assess, particularly on a long-term basis, as would be required.

Our vision is not impossibly Utopian but eminently realisable. It does not require cataclysmic changes to the established order but rather a bringing together of interests and skills that exist but today operate independently. The application of discipline and clear thinking to a new national model could provide a service which could be worthy of a new century.

REFERENCES

High Security Psychiatric Services Commissioning Board (1996/7) *Contract with Providers (Special Hospitals)*. London: HSPSCB.

Longford, Lord (1992) *Prisoner or Patient*. London: Chapmans Publishers.

SHSA (1992) *Security in the Special Hospitals*. London: SHSA.

Steels *et al.* (1997) *Discharged from Special Hospital Under Restriction*. Submitted to CBMH for publication.

Willis, J. (1995) *The Paradox of Progress*. Oxford: Radcliffe Medical Press.

Appendix 1: SHSA Patient's Charter (Summary)

When You Come Into Hospital

- Once it has been agreed that you should come into hospital, you will be given a guaranteed admission date within a maximum of three months.
- Within one hour of arriving at the hospital you will be seen by the Patient Services Manager (or his/her representative), who will tell you the name of the ward to which you have been assigned.
- The Patient Services Manager will complete part of your personal records and tell you about the hospital and the way it works.
- As soon as possible after arrival at your ward, you will be introduced to your named qualified nurse who will look after you and develop your nursing care plan with you.
- You will be seen by a doctor within 12 hours of arriving at the hospital or before 10 p.m. on the day of admission, whichever is the sooner.

While You Are In Hospital

- A named Consultant will be responsible for treating your mental disorder.
- It is your right to seek a second opinion about any aspect of your treatment for your mental disorder.
- You may request a change of Consultant.
- There is no obligation upon you to take part in the training of unqualified staff or in research.
- The hospital is committed to provide the best possible treatment available for your clinical condition.
- Your initial treatment plan will be drawn up with you within one working week of admission.
- Your treatment plan will be reviewed at a full case conference (i.e. by all members of your clinical team led by your Consultant) within six months of your admission into hospital.
- Major treatment plan reviews will take place at agreed intervals. These intervals will not be longer than 12 months.
- The treatment plan will be discussed with you at the time it is first drawn up and each time it is reviewed.
- You will be given a clear explanation of every treatment proposed in the treatment plan. Any risks and alternatives will be explained to you.
- If you are unable to give, or if you withhold, your consent to medical treatments for your mental disorder, the Mental Health Act 1983 lays down what happens next.

o If you have any disability or impediment which makes it more difficult for you to understand explanations, or if your primary language is other than English, arrangements will be made to help you understand the treatment proposed.

o While in the hospital, you will be given maximum opportunity to follow a physically healthy lifestyle.

o You will receive medical advice and all relevant physical and dental checks to promote good health.

o In the event of physical ill health, you will have access to a GP. If necessary you will be transferred to a local acute hospital for more specialised physical treatment.

o It is your right to seek a second opinion about any aspect of your physical treatment.

o You will be cared for with respect for your rights as a citizen. Certain liberties and entitlements taken for granted in the community have to be restricted while you are legally detained but this will only happen to the extent that it is necessary for your effective care and treatment, and will be discussed with you and wherever possible, your family.

o You have the right to maintain contact with and be visited by anyone you wish within certain restrictions.

o A decision to exclude any visitor is rare. Any such decision will be fully recorded and available for independent examination by the Mental Health Act Commission.

o We will honour all your legal rights as set out in the Mental Health Act 1983, the Mental Health Act Code of Practice, the Data Protection Act 1984, the Hospital Complaints Procedure Act 1985 and the Access to Health Records Act 1990.

Appendix 2: Statistics

The following tables are based on information kindly provided by Martin Butwell from the Professorial Unit at Broadmoor Hospital. They represent only a small sample from the wealth of information that the statistical unit and Case Register hold. The Professorial Unit will be publishing its own comprehensive statistical review. A few key points are worth noting:

1. The reduction in the overall resident population in the service as a whole and in each hospital (particularly at Liverpool).

2. The continuing demand expressed as referrals – higher in recent years than in the late 1980s.

3. The continuing increase in both absolute numbers and proportions of patients from ethnic minorities (mainly black Afro-Caribbean).

4. The steady reduction in the number of women patients.

5. The decline in admissions and residents of learning disability patients.

Table 1 In patient population at year end 1988–96

	Broadmoor	Rampton	Ashworth	Total
1988	519	562	653	1734
1989	504	559	652	1715
1990	494	549	648	1691
1991	486	553	646	1685
1992	486	546	625	1657
1993	481	515	600	1596
1994	475	488	554	1517
1995	471	474	543	1488
1996	476	482	501	1459

Table 2 Referrals, admissions* and departures* 1988–96

All hospital referrals		Broadmoor		Rampton		Ashworth		Totals	
		Adm.	Depart	Adm.	Depart	Adm.	Depart	Adm.	Depart
1988	316	78	41	59	70	57	76	194	187
1989	302	56	68	50	74	79	82	185	204
1990	298	36	49	58	67	77	79	171	195
1991	322	58	63	57	54	67	67	182	184
1992	335	74	72	61	70	54	74	189	216
1993	418	59	61	81	113	61	86	201	260
1994	448	70	78	56	85	45	90	171	253
1995	411	57	60	62	76	6	72	180	208
1996	N/A	56	51	82	72	150	89	188	212
		544	543	566	661	551	715	1661	1919

*Excluding inter-hospital transfers

Table 3 Gender and ethnicity 1988–96

Totals for all hospitals					Total
	Male		Female		
	Non-white	Total	Non-white	Total	
1988	198	1385	33	349	1734
1989	214	1385	30	330	1715
1990	218	1374	28	317	1691
1991	223	1387	28	298	1685
1992	224	1373	28	284	1657
1993	226	1338	26	258	1596
1994	221	1269	27	248	1517
1995	236	1256	29	232	1488
1996	240	1233	32	226	1459

Table 4: Learning disability patients:
Referrals, admissions and departures 1988–96

All hospital referrals		Ashworth		Rampton		Broadmoor		Totals	
		Adm.	Depart	Adm.	Depart	Adm.	Depart	Adm.	Depart
1988	41	5	13	11	21	–	1	16	35
1989	42	8	6	4	11	–	1	12	18
1990	30	6	7	4	10	–	–	10	17
1991	24	5	11	5	10	–	–	10	21
1992	21	2	8	3	12	–	–	5	20
1993	19	1	9	4	20	–	–	5	29
1994	17	–	8	2	16	–	–	2	24
1995	20	–	4	4	15	–	1	4	20
1996	n/a	–	9	3	11	–	–	3	20
Totals		27	75	40	126	0	3	67	204

Appendix 3: SHSA Media Guidelines

Rights of Patients

- We will protect the privacy and confidentiality of our patients.
- We will not release any information about a patient without their consent, and will involve them and their clinical teams in decisions about media access.
- If a patient is unable to give consent, we will ask a relative, close friend or other person previously nominated by them.
- If we hear that a reporter has inaccurate information about a patient which may be damaging to them, we will try to prevent its publication. If inaccurate information is published, we will consider taking further action against the publishers.
- If a patient wants to make a statement in response to inaccurate reporting we may, after considering the request together with the clinical team, help by contacting and advising a relative, friend, or other person to speak on their behalf.
- If a patient wants to speak to the media, we will consider the request carefully together with their clinical team, taking into account any adverse consequences for the patient. The interests of other patients, and the security of the hospital will also be considered. The final decision will rest with the general manager.
- If a patient withdraws his or her consent to be interviewed, or for an interview to be broadcast, we will support the patient's decision.
- If a patient is seriously injured or dies while at a special hospital we will let relatives know before details are released to the media.

Rights and Responsibilities of the Media

- We will be open in our dealings with the media.
- We will share information as fully as possible, unless it concerns a patient who has not given consent to the release of personal information, or aspects of security which could present a risk to the safe running of the hospital.
- We will delegate a member of staff, usually the public relations manager or general manager, to communicate with the media.
- We will respond to enquiries as quickly as possible.
- Requests for an interview with the patient will be considered by their psychiatrist and clinical team. It may be refused if it is not considered to be in the interests of the patient, other patients, or hospital security. The final decision will rest with the general manager.

- Journalists should only contact staff through the public relations manager or general manager.

- In the interests of our patients we will only allow taped interviews once the SHSA's broadcasting contract has been signed. In order to protect patients from adverse consequences of being recognised, identification either visually or by name will not normally be allowed.

- Journalists may only publish information about a patient they have interviewed: they must not publish comments or opinions made about other patients in the course of the interview.

- To ensure the safety and security of the hospital journalists must not identify in words, sounds or pictures any security systems or related operations.

- In the interests of all concerned, visiting journalists, photographers and film crews will be accompanied by the public relations manager or a senior manager while on site.

Rights and Responsibilities of Staff

- All patient-related information is confidential. If contacted by a journalist you should refer the call to the public relations manager or a designated senior manager. Disclosure by staff to the media of confidential patient information will be regarded as gross misconduct.

- If in the course of your work you are asked by management to speak to the press about what you do, you will be given help and advice by the public relations manager about how to go about it. The media offer us access to the public. Try to help us answer their questions as quickly and as fully as you can.

- In the interests of patient and public safety do not discuss or give details of hospital security to journalists.

- If your patient wants to make a statement to the press remember that as a hospital employee you should not act as his or her advocate. However, a member of the clinical team could contact a person the patient nominates.

- If, because of your work, you find yourself the focus of unwelcome attention from the media we will offer you help and support to deal with it.

- We will not disclose your name, address, or other personal details without your consent.

- If we hear the media intend to publish information about you which is untrue we will try to stop it. If information is published which is untrue we will consider taking action against the publishers.

The Contributors

William Bingley

William Bingley is a lawyer by training and since 1990 has been the Chief Executive of the Mental Health Act Commission. He was Legal Director of MIND (National Association for Mental Health) from 1983 to 1989 when he was seconded to the Department of Health as Executive Secretary of the Working Group preparing the Mental Health Act Code of Practice which was published in 1990. He was a member of the Secretary of State's Working Group on the Future of High Security Psychiatric Provision, is currently a co-opted member of the BMA Medical Ethics Committee and has observer status on the Law Society's Mental Health and Disability Sub-Committee.

Diana Dickens

Diana Dickens was formally Consultant in Learning Disability to Leavesden Hospital, Leavesden in the London Borough of Harrow, 1985–1993. She was firstly Medical Director and then Unit General Manager at Rampton Hospital. Since then, she has been Advisor in Forensic Psychiatry to Trent Regional Health Authority and is currently Clinical Director and Consultant in Learning Disabilities to the Department of Mental Health and Learning Disabilities, Bassetlaw District General Hospital. Other activities include extensive involvement with the Royal College of Psychiatrists, including appointments such as Chairman for the Learning Disabilities Section and Vice President member of the National Development Team for Learning Disabilities for eight years. She has also been a member of the All Wales Advisory Panel for four years.

David E. Edmond

David Edmond trained in Agriculture and Life Sciences before working for the Colonial Office in Malawi, C. Africa. After further education in the USA, he joined the Imperial Tobacco Company as Research Director in America. Later he moved with the company to Ireland and England before finally taking early retirement as head of John Player and Sons in 1986.

Since leaving the SHSA he has worked as a consultant for TEC International UK Ltd in the field of Chief Executive training and development.

Jim Higgins

Jim Higgins was a Consultant Forensic Psychiatrist in Mersey since 1975, member of the Special Hospitals Service Authority from 1989 to 1996 and a member of the Advisory Board on Restricted Patients from 1990 to 1996. He is currently a member of the High Security Psychiatric Services Commissioning Board and Honorary Clinical Lecturer in Forensic Psychiatry to the University of Liverpool.

Roger Hinton

Roger Hinton was the Special Hospitals Service Authority's Director of Capital Resources between 1990 and 1996, when he was responsible for developing and managing the Authority's capital programme. He has wide experience of the health service and especially of health planning, both in the NHS and overseas. His particular interest is the introduction of commercial practices into health service building programme management, design and construction.

Joy Kinsley OBE

Joy Kinsely trained as a nurse at St Thomas' Hospital and subsequently as a midwife. She was a district nurse/midwife in Bedfordshire for six and a half years and a Mental Welfare Officer in Bedfordshire for three and a half years. She obtained London University's External Diploma in Social Studies. In 1966 she joined the Prison Service as an Assistant Governor and remained in that service for 23 years. During that time, she gained extensive experience as a governor and held a number of senior posts, including administrative posts in the South East Region; she became Governor of Holloway Prison and subsequently Brixton Prison. In 1989 she left the Prison Service, after a period in the Prison Service Inspectorate and joined the newly formed SHSA, firstly as Head of Personnel and Director of Home Office Liaison and latterly as Director of Security. She retired from full-time work in 1992, but continued to advise the SHSA on security matters until 1995. She was a member of the Parole Board from 1992 to 1996.

Jane Mackenzie

Jane Mackenzie has almost 30 years experience in Forensic Psychiatric Health Care having trained as an RMN at Broadmoor Hospital between 1968 and 1971. She has experience in general NHS Psychiatric Services, Addictions, Challenging Behaviours, Physical Health Care, Care of the Elderly and Ward Management. She has played a significant role in the development of Quality Services at Broadmoor Hospital and is currently the Quality Improvement Services Manager. She graduated with a Master Degree in 'Quality Management in Health Care' in 1995.

David Mawson

David Mawson has worked in Broadmoor and Moss Side hospitals, in both of which he has been Medical Director. He has held similar positions in two private companies, helping to set up long-term medium secure beds. Currently he is pursuing interests outside psychiatry though continuing with Parole Board and medico-legal work.

Margaret C. Orr

After house jobs in surgery and medicine at Glasgow Victoria and Royal Infirmaries, Dr Margaret Orr began GP training in Greenock, spending part of her time at the only prison for women in Scotland. Contact with the prison continued while working in the local maternity hospital where prisoners were delivered of their babies. Over the next ten years she continued this contact while working as a psychiatric registrar in Ravenscraig Hospital, Greenock. This kindled an interest in Forensic Psychiatry which led to her becoming a senior registrar at the Wessex Regional Secure Unit at Knowle Hospital, Fareham. Following four years as a Prison Medical Officer at HMP Winchester, Dr Orr became a Consultant Forensic Psychiatrist at Broadmoor Hospital in 1988. Between 1992 and 1994 she acted as Director of Medical Services at Broadmoor and was fully appointed to that post for a further 15 months. The understanding and treatment of the patient has at all times been the fundamental principle of Margaret Orr's career.

Frank Powell

Frank Powell worked for 34 years in the NHS. He commenced by obtaining nursing qualifications in general, psychiatric and learning disability and then developed his career as a professional nurse leader. During the 1980s he served as a Chief Nursing Officer in Hertfordshire and then became Head of Nursing Services for the Special Hospitals Service Authority from its inception in 1989 until its closure. He has contributed widely to professional work at a national level. He now continues as a consultant and lecturer and works within the Independent Health Sector as Director of Nursing, Behavioural Care and Diagnostics Division, Westminster Health Care.

Pamela Taylor

Pamela Taylor is Professor of Special Hospital Psychiatry at the Institute of Psychiatry in London, and Broadmoor Hospital Authority. She has previously worked in a variety of clinical settings, but principally with offender patients in medium security or in the community. For five years from 1990 she was Head of Medical Services for the Special Hospitals Service Authority. She has also worked with victims and survivors of criminal assault and disasters. Her association with the Probation Service is long standing, and she is currently a member of the Inner London Probation Service Board. She has worked in the USA as well as the UK. Her research interests are wide, and include publications on treatments for schizophrenia; mental disorder and violence; life-sentenced prisoners; and victims and survivors of disaster, accidents or crime. She is, with John Gunn, editor of the text book *Forensic Psychiatry: Clinical, Legal and Ethical Issues*. She is editor of a book *Violence in Society*. She also co-edits with John Gunn and David Farrington the journal *Criminal Behaviour and Mental Health*.

Trevor Walt

The Reverend Trevor Walt worked as a nurse and tutor at Broadmoor Hospital for 17 years before becoming an Anglican priest. Having been appointed as a student psychiatric nurse in 1971, he qualified in 1974 and worked as a staff nurse until moving to the nurse education department. From 1983 to 1986 he underwent part-time theological training and was ordained as an Anglican priest in 1987. He has been full-time Church of England chaplain since 1988.

Glossary

BMJ	British Medical Journal
COHSE	Confederation of Heath Service Employees
DHSS	Department of Health and Social Security
DH	Department of Health
HAS	Health Advisory Service
HMT	Hospital Management Team
HSPSCB	High Security Psychiatric Services Commissioning Board
Index Offence	The criminal offence that requires a person to be detained in Special Hospital
MDO	Mentally disordered offender
MIND	The National Association for Mental Health
MHAC	Mental Health Act Commission
MLD	Mild learning disability
MSU	Medium Secure Unit
NSF	National Schizophrenia Fellowship
NUPE	Nations of Unions of Public Employees
POA	Prison Officers' Association
PSA	Property Services Agency
RCN	Royal College of Nursing
Restricted patient	A patient whose movement is restricted by the Home Office under the Mental Health Act 1983
RMNH	Registered Mental Nurse for the Handicapped
RMO	Responsible Medical Officer as defined under the Mental Health Act 1983
SANE	Schizophrenia: A National Emergency (pressure group)
SHRU	Special Hospitals research unit
SHSA	Special Hospitals Service Authority
SHSB	Special Hospitals Service Board – responsible for the Special Hospitals up to 1989
SLD	Severe learning disability
The Dutch TBS	Terbeschikkingstelling (literally 'detention at Her Majesty's pleasure')
UKCC	United Kingdom Central Council (for nursing)
UNISON	A major health service union
WISH	Women in Special Hospitals and Secure Psychiatric Units (pressure group)

Bibliography

Adams, J. (1996) *Risk*. London: UCL Press (Third Impression).

Allen, C. (1997) *Nursing Times*. 26 March.

Appelbaum, P.S. and Jorgenson, L.M. (1991) 'Psychotherapist–patient sexual contact after termination of treatment.' *American Journal of Psychiatry 148*, 1466–1473.

Ashworth Patient Advocacy Service (1994) *Ashworth Patient Advocacy Service Report*. p.2.

Ashworth Report (1992) *Report of the Committee of Inquiry into Complaints about Ashworth Hospital. 1*, p.146.

Bailey, J. and MacCullough, M. (1992) 'Patterns of reconviction in patients discharged directly to the community from a Special Hospital.' *Journal of Forensic Psychiatry 1013*, 445–461.

Barnes, R.C. and Earnshaw, S. (1993) 'Mental illness in British newspapers.' *Psychiatric Bulletin 17*, 673–674.

Bartlett, A. (1993) 'Rhetoric and reality: what do we know about the English special hospitals?' *International Journal of Law and Psychiatry 16*, 27–52.

Bingley, W. (1996) *Hospital Inquiries: Have We Learnt Anything?* London: Criminal Behaviour and Mental Health Supplement.

Bingley, W. *Hospital Inquiries – Criminal Behaviour and Mental Health*. (1995 supplement).

Blom-Cooper, L. (1992) *Report of the Committee of Inquiry into Complaints about Ashworth Hospital*. London: HMSO 2028, 1 and 2.

Blom-Cooper, L. (1993) *Current Legal Problems 46 Part 2*. OUP.

Blom-Cooper, L. *et al.* (1992) *Report of the Committee of Inquiry into Complaints about Ashworth Hospital*. London: HMSO.

HMSO (1985) *Mental Health Act Commission. First Biennial Report 1983–1985*. London: HMSO.

Blom-Cooper, L. *et al.* (1992) *Report of the Committee of Inquiry into Complaints about Ashworth Hospital*. HMSO Cm 2028–I and II.

Blumenthal, R., Kreisman, D. and O'Connor, P. (1982) 'Returned to the family and its consequence for rehospitalisation among recently discharged mental patients.' *Psychological Medicine 12*, 141–147.

Bourgeois, M. (1975) 'Sexualité et Institution Psychiatrique.' *Evolution Psychiatrique 40*, 551–573.

Boynton Report (1980) *Report of the Review of Rampton Hospital* (Cmnd 8073). London: HMSO.

Butler Committee, The (1972) *Report of the Committee on Mentally Abnormal Offenders*. (Cmnd 6224) HMSO.

Bynoe, I. (1995) 'The Falling Shadow: A Lawyer's View'. *Journal of Forensic Psychiatry 6*, 3, 588–593.

Cavior, H.E. and Cohen, S.H. (1980) 'The development of a scale to assess inmate and staff attitudes toward co-corrections.' In J.O. Smykla (ed) *Coed Prison*. New York: Human Sciences Press.

Committee on the Family, Group for the Advancement of Psychiatry (1995) 'A model for the classification and diagnosis of relational disorder.' *Psychiatric Services 46*, 926–931.

Cope, R. (1989) 'The compulsory detention of Afro-Caribbeans under the Mental Health Act.' *New Community*, 343–356.

Cox, M. and Theilgaard, A. (1987) *Mutative Metaphors in Psychotherapy*. London: Jessica Kingsley Publishers.

Criminal Behaviour and Mental Health (1992) 'Psychopathic Disorder.' *Criminal Behaviour and Mental Health 2, 2*

Day, K. (1994) 'Psychiatric services in mental retardation – genetics or specialised provision?' *Psychiatric Disorders in Mental Retardation.* Cambridge: Cambridge University Press.

Dell, S. (1980) 'Transfer of Special Hospital patients to NHS hospitals.' *British Journal of Psychiatry 136*, 222–234.

Dell, S. and Robertson, G. (1988) 'The attitudes and practices of Special Hospital consultants in relation to patients classified as psychopathically disordered.' Maudsley Monographs No.32. Oxford: OUP.

Department of Health (1989a) *Operational Brief (May).* London: DH.

Department of Health (1989b) *Policy Guidelines (October).* London: DH.

Department of Health (1993) *Services for People with Learning Disabilities & Challenging Behaviours or Mental Health Needs.* London: HMSO.

DHSS and the Welsh Office (1971) *Better Services for the Mentally Handicapped* (Cmnd 4683). London: HMSO.

Dolan, B. and Coid, J. (1993) *Psychopathic and Antisocial Personality Disorders: Treatment and Research Issues.* London: Gaskell.

Dolan, B. and Coid, J. (1993) *Psychopathic and Antisocial Personality Disorders – Treatment and Research Issues.* London: Gaskell.

Donovan, M. (1997) *Broadmoor Hospital: External Management Review.* NHS Executive: Anglia and Oxford.

Donovan Report (1997) Paras.4.8 and 12.1. Anglia and Oxford: NHS Executive.

Duggan, C. 'Couples' assessment' (in press) In P.J. Taylor and T. Swann (eds) *Couples in Care and Custody.* Butterworth Heinemann: Oxford.

Evening Post (1993) 16 December.

Feldbrugge, J.T.T.M. (Personal communication) Van der Hoer Kliniek, Postbus 174, Willem Dresslaan 2, Utrecht, Netherlands.

Fernando, S. (1995) *Mental Health in a Multi-Ethnic Society.* London: Routledge.

Ferraro, D., Kennedy, M., Leese, M. and Taylor, P.J. (in press) 'Are national principles and the care programme approach likely to be enough?'

Fitzgerald, E. and Harbour, A. (in press) 'Marriages and partnerships for psychiatric patients or prisoners: European rights and the law in England and Wales.' In P.J. Taylor and T. Swann (eds) *Couples in Care and Custody.* Butterworth Heinemann: Oxford.

Fraser, W. and Nolan, M. (1994) 'Psychiatric disorders in mental health retardation.' In Bouras , S. (ed) *Mental Health in Mental Retardation.* Cambridge: Cambridge University Press.

Gartrell, N., Herman, J., Olarte, S., Feldstein, M. and Localio, R. (1986) 'Psychiatrist–patient sexual contact: results of a national survey. I: prevalence.' *American Journal of Psychiatry 143*: 1126–1131.

Gartrell, N., Herman, J., Olarte, S., Feldstein, M. and Localio, R. (1987) 'Reporting practice of psychiatrists who knew of sexual misconduct by colleagues.' *American Journal of Psychiatry 57*, 287–296.

Goffman, E. (1968) *Asylums.* London: Pelican Press.

Gonsiorek, J.C. (ed) (1995) *Breach of Trust. Sexual Exploitation by Health Care Professionals and Clergy.* Thousand Oaks, CA: Sage.

Gordon, H. (in press) 'International perspectives on the theory and practice of sexuality in secure institutions.' In P.J. Taylor and T. Swann (eds) *Couples in Care and Custody.* Butterworth Heinemann: Oxford.

Gostin, L.O. (1977) *A Human Condition: The Law Relating to Mentally Abnormal Offenders: Observations, Analysis and Proposals for Reform.* Vol.2. London: MIND.

Grounds, A.T. (1987) 'Detention of "psychopathic disorder" patients in special hospitals: critical issues.' *British Journal of Psychiatry 151*, 474–478.

Grounds, A.T. (1997) 'Commentary on "Inquiries, who needs them"' *Psychiatric Bulletin 21*, 3, 133–134.

Häfner, H. and Böker, W. (1973), (translated by H. Marshall, 1982) *Crimes of Violence by Mentally Abnormal Offenders.* Cambridge: Cambridge University Press.

Harding, L. (1985) *Born a Number.* London: Mind.

HAS (1988) *Health Advisory Service Report on Broadmoor Hospital.* London: HAS.

Heads, T., Leese, M., Taylor, P.J. and Phillips, S. (in press) 'A special hospital sample of patients with schizophrenia: social integration, aspects of illness and violent behaviour.'

High Security Psychiatric Services Commissioning Board (1996/7) Contract with providers (Special Hospitals).

HMSO (1987) *Mental Health Act Commission. Second Biennial Report 1985–1987.* London: HMSO.

HMSO (1989) *Mental Health Act Commission. Third Biennial Report 1987–1989.* London: HMSO.

HMSO (1991) *Mental Health Act Commission. Fourth Biennial Report 1989–1991.* London: HMSO.

HMSO (1992) *Report of the Committee of Inquiry into Complaints about Ashworth Hospital.* London: HMSO.

HMSO (1993) *Mental Health Act Commission. Fifth Biennial Report 1991–1993.* London: HMSO.

HMSO (1995) *Mental Health Act Commission. Sixth Biennial Report 1993–1995.* London: HMSO.

Holbrook, T. (1989) 'Policing sexuality in a modern state hospital.' *Hospital and Community Psychiatry 40*, 75–79.

Home Office (1989) *Mentally Disordered Offenders.* London: HMSO.

Home Office (1997) *Home Office Statistical Bulletin.* Issue 20/97, September.

Home Office: Research and Statistics Department (1995) *Statistics of Mentally Disordered Offenders: 1994.* HMSO: London.

Human Rights Watch Women's Rights Project (1996) *All Too Familiar: Sexual Abuse of Women in US State Prisons.*

Hutchinson, G., Takei, N., Fahy, T.A. and Bhughra, D. (1996) 'Morbid risk of schizophrenia in first-degree relatives of white and afro-carribean patients with psychosis.' *British Journal of Psychiatry 169*, 6, 776–780.

Institute of Psychiatry and the Maudsley Hospital, Research Report 1996.

Jamison, K.R. (1996) *An Unquiet Mind.* London: Picador.

Johnson, S. (1997) *London's Mental Health.* London: King's Fund.

Kaye, C. (1998) 'Hallmarks of a secure psychiatric service for women.' *Psychiatric Bulletin 22*, 3, 137–140.

Kaye, C. and Blee, T. (eds) (1997) *The Arts in Health Care: A Palette of Possibilities.* London: Jessica Kingsley Publishers.

Kershaw, C. and Kershaw, G. (1997) *Home Office Statistical Bulletin Issue 20/97.* London: Government Statistical Service.

Knight, M. (1950) *William James.* London: Penguin.

Kohner, N. (1995) *Clinical Supervision in Practice.* London: King's Fund Centre.

Laumann, E.O., Gagnon, J.H., Michael, R.T. and Michaels, S. (1994) *The Social Organization of Sexuality: Sexual Practices in the United States.* Chicago: University of Chicago Press.

Lewis, D. (1997) *Hidden Agendas.* London: Hamish Hamilton.

Lewontin, R.C. (1995) 'Sex, lies and social science.' *The New York Review of Books XLII*, 24–29.

Longford, Lord (1992) *Prisoner or Patient.* London: Chapmans Publishers.

Low, G., Terry, G. and Duggan, C. (in press) 'Deliberate self harm among female patients at a special hospital.' *Health Trends 29*, 1, 6–9.

Maden, A., Curle, C., Meux, C., Burrows, S. and Gunn, J. (1995) *Treatment and Security Needs of Special Hospital Patients*. London: Whurr Publishers.

Martin, J. (1984) *Hospitals in Trouble*. Oxford: Basil Blackwell.

Mason, T. (1993) Seclusion *Theory Reviewed, Medicine, Science and the Law 33*, 95–102.

Mawson, D.C. (1983) '"Psychopaths" in special hospitals.' *Bulletin of the Royal College of Psychiatrists 7*, 178–181.

Merikangas (1982) 'Assortive mating for psychiatric disorders and psychological traits.' *Archives of General Psychiatry 39*, 173–1180.

Meux, C. (1995) 'Management for dangerous mentally disordered prisoners in England and Wales.' *Criminal Behaviour and Mental Health 5*, 1, 3–8.

Miller, L.J. and Finnerty, M. (1996) 'Sexuality, pregnancy, and child rearing among women with schizophrenia-spectrum disorders.' *Psychiatric Services 47*, 502–506.

Monahan, J. and Steadman, H.J. (eds) (1994) *Violence and Mental Disorder (Developments in Risk Assessment)*. Chicago: University of Chicago Press.

Muijen, M. (1997) 'Inquiries, who needs them?' *Psychiatric Bulletin 21*, 3, 132–133.

Mullen, P. (1996) *Criminal Behaviour and Mental Health*. Vol.6, No.1, p.40.

Mulligan, T. and Moss, C.R. (1991) 'Sexuality and aging in male veterans: a cross-sectional study of interest, ability and activity.' *Archives of Sexual Behavior 20*, 17–25.

Murphy, E. (1977) 'The future of Britain's high security hospitals.' *British Medical Journal 314*, 1292–1293.

Murphy, E. (1996) 'The past and future of special hospitals.' *Journal of Mental Health 5*, 5, 475–482.

Murphy, E. (1997) 'The future of Britains high security hospitals.' (Editorial) *BMJ* No. 7090 3 May.

Nacci, P.L. and Kane, T.R. (1984) 'Sex and sexual aggression in federal prisons: inmate involvement and employee impact.' *Federal Probation 40*, 46–53.

Nature (1996) 27 March, p.310.

NHS and DHSS (1988) *Report on the Services Provided by Broadmoor Hospital*. NHS HAS and DHSS SSI.

NHS Executive (1997) *Ethics Committee Review of Multi-Centre Research – HSG(97)32*. NHS Executive.

NHS Health Advisory Service (1988) *Report on Broadmoor Hospital*. London: HAS 551(88), SH1.

NHS Health Advisory Service (1995) *With Care in Mind*. London: NHS/HAS.

Nursing Times, 93, 2, 8 January.

Openmind (1990/1991) No.48 (Dec 1990/Jan 1991) p.30.

Parnas, J. (1985) 'Mates of schizophrenic mothers; a study of assortative mating from the American–Danish High Risk Project.' *British Journal of Psychiatry 146*, 490–497.

Peary, J. (1996) *Inquiries after Homicide*. London: Duckworth.

Pfeiffer, E., Verwerdt, A. and Wang, H.S. (1969) 'The natural history of sexual behaviour in a biologically advantaged group of aged individuals.' *Journal of Gerontology 24*, 193–198.

Philo, G. (1996) *Media and Mental Distress*. London: Longman.

Pilgrim, D. (1990/1991) In Openmind No.48, December 1990/January 1991.

Planansky, K. and Johnston, R. (1977) 'Homicidal aggression in schizophrenic men.' *Acta Psychiatrica Scandinavica 55*, 65–73.

Porter, R. (1989) *A Social History of Madness*. London: Weidenfeld and Nicolson.

Powell, F. *et al.* (1993) *Evaluation of the Impact of Ward Managers in their First Year of Appointment*. London: SHSA.

Prins, H. (1995) *Offenders, Deviants or Patients?* London: Routledge (2nd Edition).

Proceedings of Conference held in Nottingham. (January 1996) *Schizophrenia – Current Advances in Research and Treatment.* SHSA and Rampton Hospital.

Rampton Hospital Council (1994) *Second Annual Report (Sept 93–June 94).* Retford: RHC.

Reading Evening Standard (1996) 28 November.

Reason, J. (1990) *Human Error.* Cambridge: Cambridge University Press.

Reder, P. and Duncan, S. (1996) 'Inquiries After Homicide'. Edited by J. Peary. *Inquiries After Homicide.* London: Duckworth.

Reed (1994) 'Review of Health and Social Services for Mentally Disordered Offenders and others requiring similar services' Vol.7. *People with Learning Disabilities (Mental Handicap) or with Autism.* London: HMSO.

Report concerning the death of Michael Martin (The Ritchie Report) (1985)

Robinson, D.N. (1996) *Wild Beasts and Idle Humours.* London: Harvard University Press.

Rutherford, A. (1996) *Transforming Criminal Policy.* Winchester: Waterside Press.

Ryan, N. (1996) *Lobbying from Below.* London: UCL Press.

Salokangas, R.K.R. (1983) 'Prognostic implications of the sex of schizophrenic patients.' *British Journal of Psychiatry 142,* 145–151.

Sandford, T. and Courtney, K. (1996) *Perspectives in Mental Health Nursing.* London: Baillière Tindall.

Schweber, C. (1984) 'Beauty marks and blemishes: the coed prison as a microcosm of integrated society.' *Prison Journal 64,* 3–14.

Scull, A.T. (1979) *Museums of Madness.* London: Allen Lane Penguin Books.

Shanks, J. and Atkins, P. (1985) 'Psychiatric patients who marry each other.' *Psychological Medicine 15,* 377–382.

Sheppard, D. (1995) *Learning the Lessons.* London: The Zito Trust.

SHRU (1977) *Special Hospitals Case Register – The First Five Year.* SHRU.

SHSA (1989) *Policy Guidelines.* London: Department of Health.

SHSA (1989) *Prejudice and Pride.* London: SHSA.

SHSA (1990) *Inquiry into the Death of Joseph Watts.* London: SHSA.

SHSA (1991) *Nursing in Special Hospitals.* London: SHSA.

SHSA (1992) *Guidance on Action Following the Death of a Patient.* London: SHSA.

SHSA (1992) *Security in the Special Hospitals.* London: SHSA.

SHSA (1992) *SHSA Ward Design Guide.* London: SHSA.

SHSA (1993) *Big, Black and Dangerous?* London: SHSA.

SHSA (1993) *Evaluation of Impact of Ward Managers in their First Year of Appointment.* London: SHSA.

SHSA (1995) *Suicide Preventative Measures: Design Guidelines and Checklist.* London: SHSA.

Skynner, R. (1980) 'Recent developments in marital therapy.' *The Journal of Family Therapy 2,* 271–296.

Steels *et al.* (1997) *Discharged from Special Hospital Under Restriction.* Submitted to CBMH for publication.

Stevens, B.C. (1969) *Marriage and Fertility of Women Suffering from Schizophrenia or Affective Disorders.* Maudsley Monograph, No. 19. London: Oxford University Press.

Stewart, R. (1989) *Leading in the NHS.* London: Macmillan.

Swinton, M. and Hopkins, R. (1996) 'Violence and self injury.' *Journal of Forensic Psychiatry 7,* 3, 563–9.

Swinton, M. and Smith, S. (1997) 'Costs of physical health care for self injuring patients.' *Psychiatric Bulletin 21,* 9.

Taylor, P.J. (1991) *Research Strategy for the Special Hospitals, Feb 1991.* Unpublished report to SHSA.

Taylor, P. (1997) 'Clinical Research and Forensic Psychiatry.' Delivered to the Cropwood Conference, March.

Taylor, P.J., Leese, M., Williams, D., Butwell, M., Daly, R. and Larkin, E. (in press) 'Mental disorder and violence: a special hospital study.' *British Journal of Psychiatry.*

Taylor, P.J., Leese, M., Williams, D., Butwell, M., Daly, R., Larkin, E. and others in the Special Hospitals' Treatment Resistant Schizophrenia Group Mental Disorder and Violence: A Special Hospital Study. (Submitted for publication to the *British Journal of Psychiatry*).

Test, M.A., Burke, S.S. and Wallischls (1990) 'Gender differences of young adults with schizophrenic disorders in community care.' *Schizophrenia Bulletin 16,* 331–344.

The Mail on Sunday (1997) Editorial, 23 February.

The Special Hospitals Treatment Resistant Schizophrenia Research Group (1997) 'Schizophrenia violence, clozapine and risperidone: a review.' *British Journal of Psychiatry* (suppl.31) 21–30.

The Times (1995) 17 October.

Thomas, J.E. (1972) *The English Prison Officer Since 1850.* London: Routledge and Kegan Paul.

Tyrer, P. and Stein, G. (1993) *Personality Disorder Reviewed.* London: Gaskell.

Vaughan, P.J. and Badger, D. (1995) *Working with the Mentally Disordered Offender in the Community.* London: Chapman and Hall.

Walker, N. (1996) *Dangerous People.* London: Blackstone Press Ltd.

West, D.J. (1982) *Delinquency, its Roots Carers and Prospects.* London: Heinemann.

Wharton, E. (1920) *The Age of Innocence Now.* Dent: London.

WHO (1992) *The ICD-10 Classification of Mental and Behavioural Disorders.* World Health Organisation: Geneva.

WHO (1995) *The Committee on the Family.* World Health Organisation: Geneva.

Williamson, G. (1995) *Positive Press: July 1994 – July 1995.* Ashworth Hospital.

Willis, J. (1995) *The Paradox of Progress.* Oxford: Radcliffe Medical Press.

Wing, L. (1994) 'The autistic continuum Chapter 1D psychiatric disorder in mental retardation.' In Bouras (ed) *Mental Health in Mental Retardation.* Cambridge: Cambridge University Press.

Wood, J. (1995) 'Foreword.' In H. Prins *Offenders, Deviants or Patients?* Second edition. London: Routledge.

Index